The
Low-GL
Diet
Made Easy

SUCCESS STORIES USING THE HOLFORD LOW-GL DIET

I have tried dieting in the past but tend to lose interest after a few weeks, normally giving in to my sugar cravings. However, I have stuck with the Holford diet with very little need for strong willpower ... As well as losing weight I have much more energy and never feel tired during the day. Weight Loss: 11lb (5kg) in eight weeks **MF**

As a result of health problems eight months before I started the programme, I had been advised by my doctor to lose about 28lb (13kg) in weight ... The Holford programme has enabled me to lose weight in only eight weeks with little change to my diet and eating habits, and no change to my exercise routine. An added benefit was that I did not feel hungry and I did not crave any foods over the eight–week programme ... I have also seen an improvement in my cholesterol, homocysteine and blood sugar levels, and as a consequence I have been fully discharged by my hospital consultant. Weight Loss: 17.5lb (8kg) in eight weeks **TS**

I have always lost weight quite quickly on previous programmes but it always crept back on. I feel like my mindset has changed with the Holford GL diet and that it has made me realise that the changes I make need to be lifelong changes. As well losing weight I have seen a definite improvement in my mood – now my kids have their fun and happy mum back. Being organised, planning and preparing weekly meals has been, and is still my biggest challenge. I found it quite easy to give up the stimulants (I'm still working on giving up chocolate, though). I have enjoyed trying and discovering new and alternative products. Overall my skin seems clearer, my eyes brighter and I definitely feel more calm and in control of my moods. This has been the kick up the behind I needed to change my life and my future. Weight Loss: 11lb (5kg) in eight weeks **VR**

"I have had no problem keeping to the food plan, although I found reducing my alcohol intake and switching to decaf tea and coffee a challenge. I have enjoyed the whole experience – I have loads of energy and wake refreshed, I no longer suffer from constipation and my skin looks so much healthier. Weight Loss: 15lb (7kg) in eight weeks **SW**"

"I have been a consistent yo-yo dieter suffering as a consequence from low energy and being overweight. Having been on the Holford GL diet for eight weeks I have experienced sustained weight loss and improved energy ... I have better skin and my family's health has also improved – my husband has also lost weight as a result of the change to our family eating patterns. Weight Loss: 11lb (5kg) in eight weeks **JH**"

"I've lost 16 pounds in six weeks. My blood sugar is well under control (I'm diabetic) and I've been able to halve my medication. It's been so easy. I have no cravings. Weight Loss: 16lb (7kg) in six weeks **LB**"

"I lost 10lb (4.5kg) in five weeks, never felt hungry, I slept better, had more energy, my skin improved dramatically. I haven't put the weight back on and I still feel amazing. Weight Loss: 10lb (4.5kg) in five weeks **GS**"

"After having felt constantly tired and run down, I started the Holford GL diet. During the first month I followed the diet very strictly ... I was delighted to have lost a stone (6kg) in weight within the first four weeks ... Now I feel great – I no longer rely on cups of tea and sweet foods to keep me going. I am continuing to follow the Holford GL diet and definitely recommend it. Weight Loss: 17lb (8kg) in eight weeks **SC**"

ALSO PUBLISHED BY PIATKUS

Other Low-GL Diet titles by Patrick Holford:
The Low-GL Diet Bible
The Low-GL Diet Cookbook (recipes by Fiona McDonald Joyce)
The Holford Diet GL Counter

Other health and nutrition titles by Patrick Holford:
100% Health
500 Top Health and Nutrition Questions Answered
Balancing Hormones Naturally (with Kate Neil)
Beat Stress and Fatigue
Boost Your Immune System (with Jennifer Meek)
Food GLorious Food (with Fiona McDonald Joyce)
Hidden Food Allergies (with Dr James Braly)
How to Quit Without Feeling S**t
    (with David Miller and Dr James Braly)
Improve Your Digestion
Natural Chill Highs
Natural Energy Highs
Natural Highs (with Dr Hyla Cass)
Optimum Nutrition Before, During and After Pregnancy
    (with Susannah Lawson)
Optimum Nutrition for the Mind
Optimum Nutrition for Your Child (with Deborah Colson)
Optimum Nutrition for Your Child's Mind (with Deborah Colson)
Optimum Nutrition Made Easy
Say No to Arthritis
Say No to Cancer
Say No to Heart Disease
Six Weeks to Superhealth
Smart Food for Smart Kids (with Fiona McDonald Joyce)
Solve Your Skin Problems (with Natalie Savona)
The Alzheimer's Prevention Plan
    (with Shane Heaton and Deborah Colson)
The Fatburner Diet
The H Factor (with Dr James Braly)
The Holford 9-day Liver Detox (with Fiona McDonald Joyce)
The Little Book of Optimum Nutrition
The Optimum Nutrition Bible
The Optimum Nutrition Cookbook (with Judy Ridgway)

patrick
HOLFORD

The
Low-GL
Diet
Made Easy

piatkus

PIATKUS

First published in Great Britain in 2006 as
The Holford Low-GL Diet Made Easy by Piatkus Books
Reprinted 2007 (three times)
Reprinted 2009 as *The Low-GL Diet Made Easy*

A CIP catalogue record for this book
is available from the British Library

ISBN 978-0-7499-2714-1

Data manipulation and typesetting by
Phoenix Photosetting, Chatham, Kent
www.phoenixphotosetting.co.uk
Printed in Italy by L.E.G.O. SpA

This book has been printed on paper manufactured
with respect for the environment using wood from
managed sustainable resources

Piatkus
An imprint of
Little, Brown Book Group
100 Victoria Embankment
London EC4Y 0DY

An Hachette UK Company
www.hachette.co.uk

www.piatkus.co.uk

CONTENTS

ACKNOWLEDGEMENTS

I'm continually learning from readers like you about what works well, and would like to thank all those early volunteers who've helped shape and prove my low-GL diet. My sincere thanks go to Sarah Sutton for her excellent editing and all the team at Piatkus for their support and attention to detail. In particular, I would like to thank Fiona McDonald Joyce for her wonderful recipes. Fiona is a qualified nutritional therapist and offers corporate consultancy on workplace nutrition as well as menu design and recipe development services. She can be contacted via fmcdj@hotmail.com.

PREFACE

I don't think of the Holford Low-GL Diet as a diet – for me it is just absolutely the best way to eat, and I will continue to eat like this for the rest of my life. Margot (44)

HOW WOULD YOU KNOW IF YOU WERE 100 PER CENT HEALTHY?

Imagine how it would feel to wake up in the morning and to leap out of bed feeling full of energy and drive. You look in the mirror and see your face with healthy-looking skin and sparkling eyes. You feel energetic, comfortable with your weight and with your body, and have no signs of exhaustion, moodiness, depression, bloating, or other 21st-century symptoms. You enjoy a delicious breakfast, and are ready to face the day. You look and feel great.

FROM TODAY...
...you will discover an easy way to lose weight, permanently

If you are suspicious of new diet claims and wary of cranky diets that involve strange eating habits and the exclusion of major food groups, you will discover from the moment you begin to read this book that the low-GL approach is easy, healthy, delicious, and, most importantly, encourages you to eat a balanced diet at all times.

WITHIN THREE DAYS...
...you will start to feel more energetic and relaxed

If you are suffering from a range of health problems that are leaving you feeling tired, run down, depressed, allergic, bloated and prematurely old, you will discover a new lease of life within three days.

> **My husband and I started the diet last Tuesday week. I have already lost 9lb (4kg) and my husband has lost 6¹/₂lb (3kg). We're both thrilled with the quick results.** Jean and Tom, early fifties

What is the reason for this apparent miracle? It is simply keeping your blood sugar balanced and your food choices healthy. The GL, or Glycemic Load – measured in GLs, of a food or meal tells you exactly what it's going to do to your blood sugar – and hence, to your weight and energy levels.

WITHIN SEVEN DAYS ...
... you will start to lose pounds as quickly as you'll gain energy

If you are one of the many people who has spent a small fortune on new diet regimes and 'miracle' foods over the years, with disappointing results, or one of the hundreds of thousands who feels disillusioned with weight-loss diets, because there is little sign of permanent success, you will realise within seven days that the Holford Low-GL Diet is different. It works with your body for optimum health as well as weight loss, so you won't even realise you are dieting.

IN JUST THREE WEEKS ...
... you will feel close to 100 per cent healthy

The Holford Low-GL Diet is a diet for the way you live today. The recipes take special account of eating on the run and the dilemmas that you may face when eating out or entertaining.

And you are not alone. By embarking on your new healthy, weight-loss path, you will be joining a community of other people with the same aims and challenges as yourself. You can get instant access to further, up-to-the minute information and advice via my website, and those who would like some moral support in a class can join one of my healthy weight-loss classes. See Further Resources (p154) for more details.

100 PER CENT HEALTH AND A DIET FOR LIFE

This book is the result of over 20 years' research in the field of diet and nutrition. The low-GL system and the easy rules explained in this book have been tried and tested around the world. The proof is in the results – and in my clients' testimonials. *The Low-GL Diet Made Easy* changes lives for the better – and provides the best permanent weight-loss solution as well. At its root are five very simple principles, which I will explain in Chapter 1.

I do all the thinking for you in the first three weeks of the diet. In the chapters that follow I will explain what 'low GL' means, how and why the low-GL system works, and how to plan for success. You will learn how to set goals, how to get started, and how to keep yourself on track.

The Low-GL Diet Made Easy is for those who want an easy-to-follow, step-by-step approach to successful weight loss that delivers plenty of fast and easy recipes with the minimum of science. Those who want more facts, figures and in-depth information about the nutritional research that underpins the diet will find *The Low-GL Diet* a useful companion volume.

You will never feel hungry on the Holford Low-GL Diet. The range of simple and flavoursome recipes created by Fiona McDonald Joyce will ensure that each meal will help you lose weight and then maintain your weight loss with ease. Fiona is a trained nutritional therapist and cook. Co-author of the bestselling book *The Low-GL Diet Cookbook*, she specialises in healthy recipes that are quick, easy and delicious.

The Holford Low-GL Diet is called 'made easy' for a reason: it is easy to understand and easy to follow. Here you will find three weeks of weight-loss menus and each recipe includes guidelines on how to adapt the recipes to maintain your weight loss. Throughout the book you will find useful fact boxes, food and preparation tips as well as recommendations from those who have used the diet successfully.

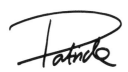

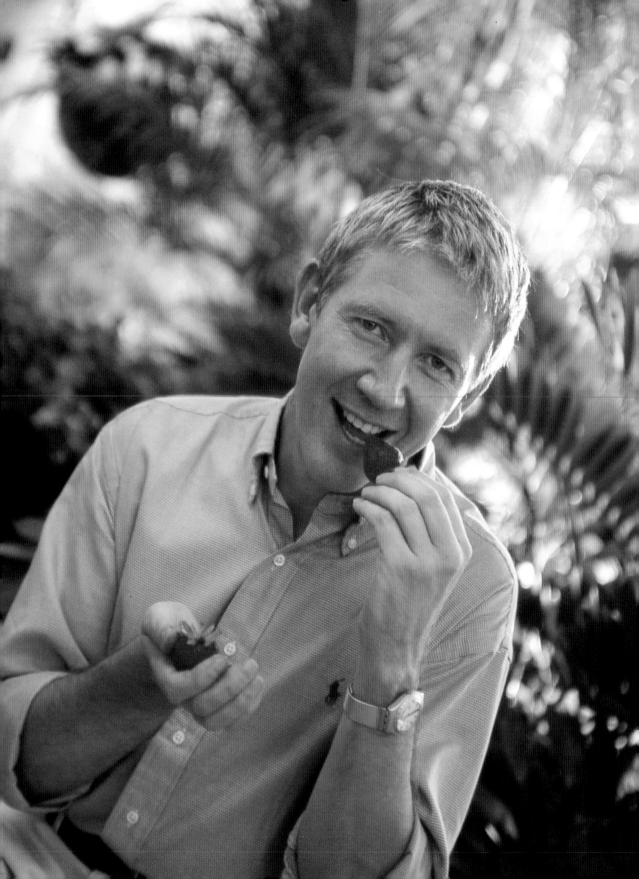

INTRODUCTION: WEIGHT LOSS MADE EASY

In Part One I will explain the five basic principles of the low-GL approach to weight loss, but first let me explain why we put on weight in the first place, what low-GL is all about, and how and why the diet works.

LOW-GL: THE PERMANENT WEIGHT-LOSS SOLUTION

The low-GL diet is the easy way to achieve healthy eating, nutrition and weight loss. It is designed as a diet for life.

WHY WE GET FAT

Have you been trying to lose weight for some time? If so, you will already know how hard it is to stay on a low-calorie diet, and will know that low-calorie diets don't lead to permanent weight loss. Low-calorie diets don't work because your body doesn't run on calories – your body operates on glucose, which it needs for energy (just as a car needs fuel). Glucose is released from your food and is then carried by blood to the cells of your body, which is why it is also called 'blood sugar'.

Your body doesn't run on calories, it runs on glucose – and it gets that glucose from your food.

Your body gets glucose mainly from the starchy foods known as carbohydrates. The best sources are vegetables, grains, sugars and fruits. When you eat more food than you need, you produce more glucose than your body can use straightaway, and so the extra is stored and turned into fat. In order to lose weight, you need to reduce your glucose levels and to start to burn off unwanted fat. That's where the Holford Low-GL Diet comes in. The diet works by making sure that you never have more glucose than your body needs, and there is never any extra glucose to turn into fat.

The Holford Low-GL Diet makes sure you never have more glucose than you need – so there will be no extra to store as fat.

Sounds too good to be true? It's time to explain what low-GL means and how the diet works.

WHAT LOW-GL MEANS AND HOW IT AFFECTS WEIGHT LOSS

GL is short for 'Glycemic (gly-see-mic) Load' and it is a unit of measurement, rather as pounds or kilos and calories are. In the Holford Low-GL Diet, GL are used to measure the amount of sugar and starch in food and their impact on the body. They show:

⇢ How much carbohydrate there is in each food (and therefore how much glucose it will create and release into the bloodstream as blood sugar).
⇢ How fast the carbohydrate will break down into glucose (and therefore how quickly your blood sugar levels will rise).

The GL of a food measures
Quantity of Carbohydrate x Quality of Carbohydrate

GL take the place of calories and other measurement systems in menu planning. In most weight-loss systems you measure calories, which tells you how much energy you need to burn off the fat you have created. The simpler GL system, however, warns you in advance how much carbohydrate there is in each meal or type of food, and what it will do to your blood sugar level – so you won't lay down the fat in the first place. This information is important because blood sugar levels are linked to hunger and the way we eat.

When you haven't eaten for a while, your blood sugar level will dip, and you will become hungry. When you eat a food containing carbohydrate, glucose is released into your bloodstream and your blood sugar level will rise again. The key to achieving your perfect weight is to keep your blood sugar levels stable. To do this you need to eat healthy foods that provide you with glucose in the right quantities.

The Holford Low-GL Diet divides carbohydrate and other foods into three levels of GL: low, medium and high. Fat-forming foods are those that cause your blood sugar to rise too fast and too high – they are the high- and medium-GL foods. The healthiest foods are the ones that take the longest to turn into glucose; that is the low-GL foods.

The secret weapon for healthy weight loss comes in the form of low-GL foods.

WHY THE HOLFORD LOW-GL DIET IS BETTER THAN THE GI DIETS

Whereas GL stands for Glycemic *Load*, GI stands for Glycemic *Index*. The Glycemic Index is a scale of measurement that tells you how fast the sugar content of a food is released into your bloodstream. GI diets (where foods are scored in line with the Glycemic Index) have enjoyed mainstream popularity in recent years and the good news is that if you have been following a GI diet you are part-way towards using the GL approach. When you follow a GI diet you use a chart that scores foods on a range from 1–100. A high GI score indicates foods to avoid; a low GI score the ones to eat. However, GI food scores, while useful, will provide only half the GL picture.

The problem is that GI doesn't tell you the quantity of the carbohydrate in the food, and so a GI food score on its own is only half the story. It is not just *how fast* the carbohydrate in your diet enters your bloodstream that it is important, it is *how much* of the food is carbohydrate. GL measure both. Take watermelon, for example: it contains fast-releasing carbohydrate. Hence it has a high GI score of 72. However, only 1/8oz (6g) per 3 1/2oz (100g) watermelon is carbohydrate. The rest of the fruit is mainly water. So the impact of the fast-releasing sugar is very low, and it has a low GL score of 4.

GL vary according to portion size, but range typically from 0–35:
Low-GL A GL of 0–10 is good
Medium-GL A GL of 11–14 is OK in moderation
High-GL A GL of 15 or more is bad, and to be avoided

The GL score of watermelon is calculated as:

$$\frac{72 \times 6 = 4.32}{100}$$

(rounded down = 4 GL)

You don't have to worry about calculations, just follow the meal planning guidelines in Chapters 6 and 7. For those who want to develop their own recipes, an up-to-date list of individual foods and their GL scores is provided on my website www.holforddiet.com and in *The Holford Diet GL Counter*.

If you keep to the low-GL guidelines:
⇢ You will stop producing more glucose than you can use.
⇢ You won't suffer from food cravings.
⇢ Your body will be reprogrammed to burn fat rapidly.
⇢ You will be able to lose weight and sustain your weight loss permanently.

THE GOOD, THE BAD AND THE UGLY

Low-GL foods are the good guys because the glucose is released into the bloodstream slowly, and blood sugar therefore remains stable. Why is that important? Because maintaining blood sugar at a stable level is the key to steady long-term weight loss. Keeping blood sugar steady prevents the energy slumps that trigger food cravings. Instead, you will develop a healthy, balanced appetite. It means your body is able to use the glucose at the same rate (or faster) than it is released, and so has none left over to store as fat.

⇢ Examples include: oatcakes, wholemeal bread, baked beans, wholemeal pasta, all vegetables (except for potatoes and parsnips), fish, white meat, eggs, soya products, milk.

Medium-GL foods are healthy in moderation. They release glucose into the bloodstream at a slower rate than high-GL foods, but still raise blood sugar to a level where it is more likely to overproduce glucose, and some will still be turned into fat. If you want to lose weight they should be limited and eaten alongside low-GL foods.

⇢ Examples include: rye crispbread, rice noodles, parsnips, boiled potatoes, bananas, rice milk.

High-GL foods are the real uglies, and are to be avoided because they release glucose into the bloodstream fast, and raise blood sugar levels too quickly for the body to cope. The body cannot use all the glucose produced and deposits a large proportion of glucose for storage as fat. Your blood sugar level then crashes – leaving you hungry again (and so the cycle continues). High-GL foods lead to food cravings that make healthy eating impossible.

⇢ Examples include: white baguette, muffins, cornflakes, all rice (except for brown basmati), couscous, puffed-rice cakes, all potatoes (except boiled), honey.

HOW THE LOW-GL DIET WORKS

You may be wondering how the Holford Low-GL Diet works and what evidence there is that it does indeed work.

There is a wealth of evidence to support the positive benefits of a low-GL diet. In the most recent study 20 people were placed on the Holford Low-GL Diet, plus basic supplements (a multivitamin, extra vitamin C and omega 3 and 6 fats) for eight weeks. Four were unable to complete for personal reasons, leaving 16. The average weight loss was a highly significant 10.25lb (4½kg), equivalent to 1.3lb (½kg) per person per week. Body fat percentage dropped by an average of 2 per cent. In addition, 94 per cent reported greater energy, 67 per cent had greater concentration, memory or alertness, 67 per cent had less indigestion or bloating, clearer and less dry skin, 50 per cent reported fewer feelings of depression and more stable moods. There was also a significant drop in blood pressure. (Holford et al. *Journal of Orthomolecular Medicine* Vol. 21, No. 2, 2006.)

But don't just take my word for it. A recent trial, published last year by the American Medical Association, compared four different diets, from conventional low-fat, high-carbohydrate diets to high-protein, low-carb diets. Of all the diets more people on a low-GL diet achieved their weight loss, and lost more fat, and had the best reduction in cardiovascular risk. The 'perfect diet' was almost identical to the Holford Low-GL Diet. (J McMillan–Price et al., 'Comparison of 4 Diets of Varying Glycemic Load', *Archives of Internal Medicine*, Vol. 166 (2006), pp. 1466–1475.)

LOW-GL AND YOUR METABOLISM

The Holford Low-GL Diet works because, on a low-GL diet, you will burn more fat than on a low-fat, low-calorie diet. That's a big statement. 'How can it be possible?' you may be thinking. The answer lies in your metabolic rate.

When you turn food into glucose, or store it as fat, you use your body's metabolism. The speed of your metabolism is known as your metabolic rate. It is partly inherited, but is linked mainly to what you eat and how active you are. The speed of your metabolism changes depending on the level of blood sugar in your body. The faster your metabolism, the faster you lose weight.

Your body needs a certain level of blood sugar to stay alive. A low-calorie diet produces very little blood sugar, which makes your body feel under threat. Your body then tries harder to hang on to blood sugar by slowing down your metabolic rate. When your metabolic rate slows down, your weight loss slows down, too, which is why, on a low-calorie diet, it becomes more and more difficult to lose weight.

On the low-GL diet, regular GL-controlled meals keep your blood sugar level stable, so your metabolic rate doesn't need to switch to survival mode. Because your metabolic rate doesn't slow down, weight loss will continue at a healthy rate. You start to feed your body fast-burn foods that don't turn into fat, which means the body can use the energy fast, and then get down to the business of burning off existing fat more rapidly.

On a low-GL diet:

⇢ You will never turn glucose into fat, so you will never gain more fat.
⇢ Your metabolism will not go into starvation or survival mode, and so it will continue to help you to burn the fat that you have.

Foods with a low GL rating encourage the body to burn fat.

THE IMPORTANCE OF EXERCISE

Exercise is the fastest way to improve your metabolic rate. Exercise also helps you to overcome fatigue, which is a common health complaint, especially among those who are overweight. Combining low-GL eating with regular exercise is important for success on the diet. This is an essential point.

I often find that when I ask people whether they exercise, the answer is 'No'. When I ask, 'Why not?' the answer is invariably, 'I'm too tired.' The instant benefit of low-GL eating is that you will have much more energy. Once you have more energy, you'll want to say 'Yes' to exercise. On a low-GL diet you will change from making fat to burning fat. (See page 55 for more about the positive benefits.)

WHY LOW-GL EATING IS BEST FOR YOUR HEALTH

Some of the most popular so-called weight-loss diets have no basis in science whatsoever, so it is not surprising when they fail in the long term. Also, many lead to a life of yo-yo dieting (repeatedly losing and gaining weight) and long-term health problems. The good results are rarely lasting. You can lose weight on a low-calorie diet, a high-protein diet, a low-carb diet or a no-fat diet, but the odds are stacked against long-term permanent success.

Why? Because:

⇢ Your body can safely burn only 2lb (1kg) of fat in a week. After that it will go into starvation mode and draw energy from lean body tissue.
⇢ A restricted diet will not fully satisfy your appetite, so you have to fight hard to stay on track.
⇢ A highly restrictive diet is unhealthy – we were not designed to live without carbohydrates or fats.

In contrast, years of research have provided evidence to prove that a low-GL diet, which combines low-GL carbohydrates with protein and essential fats, is best for optimum health and long-term weight loss.

By eating low-GL foods little and often you will reduce your calorie intake and reduce your appetite; your body will feel fully satisfied and you will suffer no cravings brought on by low blood sugar. This is why the low-GL diet recommends eating three meals and two substantial snacks a day, to a total of 40 ⓖⓛ while keeping drinks and/or desserts to a total of 5 ⓖⓛ .

On the low-GL diet you are likely to lose 6–10lb (2.7–4.5kg) a month, 2 stone/28lb (12.7kg) in three months, 8 stone/112lb (50.8kg) in a year – if you have that much to lose – with no rebound weight gain. You will lose weight steadily, moderately, healthily and, most importantly of all, permanently.

WEIGHT LOSS – FAT FACTS

⇢ You cannot lose more than 2lb (1kg) of actual fat a week unless you are starving yourself or running a marathon. You can, however, lose extra lb of excess water retention when you eat on the Holford Low-GL diet.

⇢ You can lose 7lb (3.2kg) or more fast – and permanently – if you avoid foods you are allergic to.

⇢ Losing inches is more important than losing pounds. Gaining lean body mass and losing fat are the real goals.

⇢ The body will naturally gravitate to its own ideal weight if you give it the right balance and kinds of protein, fat and carbohydrate.

There are two essential guidelines to remember for the weight-loss diet:

1 Keep your food intake to foods that total 40 ⓖⓛ a day.
2 Keep your drinks and/or desserts to 5 ⓖⓛ a day.

The good news is: the recipes in Chapter 7 will measure the units for you, but first I will explain the principles of the diet.

The benefits of the Holford Low-GL Diet

→ **You will never feel hungry** If a diet leaves you feeling famished, you won't stick to it, so from day one the low-GL diet recommends foods scientifically proven to satisfy your appetite.

→ **It's enjoyable and delicious** No food groups are excluded on the low-GL diet. You'll be able to eat bread and pasta, mayonnaise, meat – the lot. You'll just pay more attention to quality and the quantity you eat.

→ **It's safe and it's healthy** I'm not interested in helping people lose weight by cheating the body. The only side effect I want you to experience is added health.

→ **It makes you feel great** The diet works *with* your body, not against it. Your energy will increase, your mood and concentration will improve, and your skin will start to glow, within days.

→ **There will be no rebound weight gain** You are not restricting food intake and you are not suppressing your appetite. Instead you will be speeding up your metabolism – healthily – so there will be no reason for the body to store excess fat.

→ **It's easy to follow** If a diet feels easy and natural you'll stick to it for life.

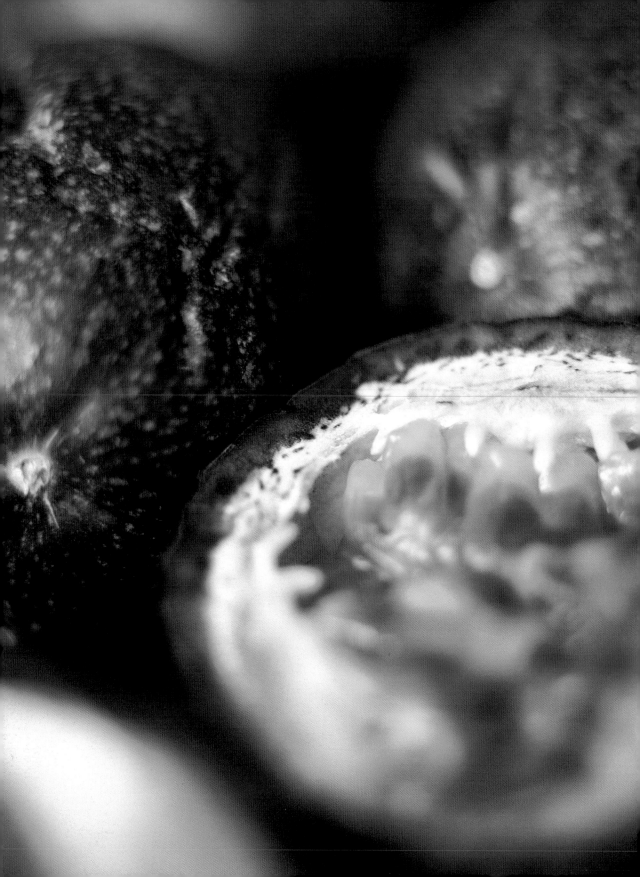

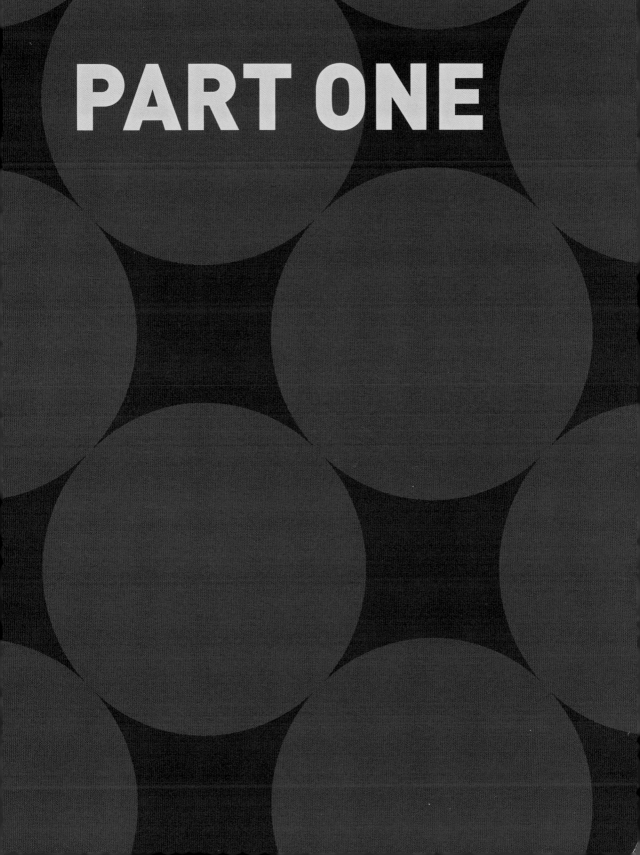

PART ONE

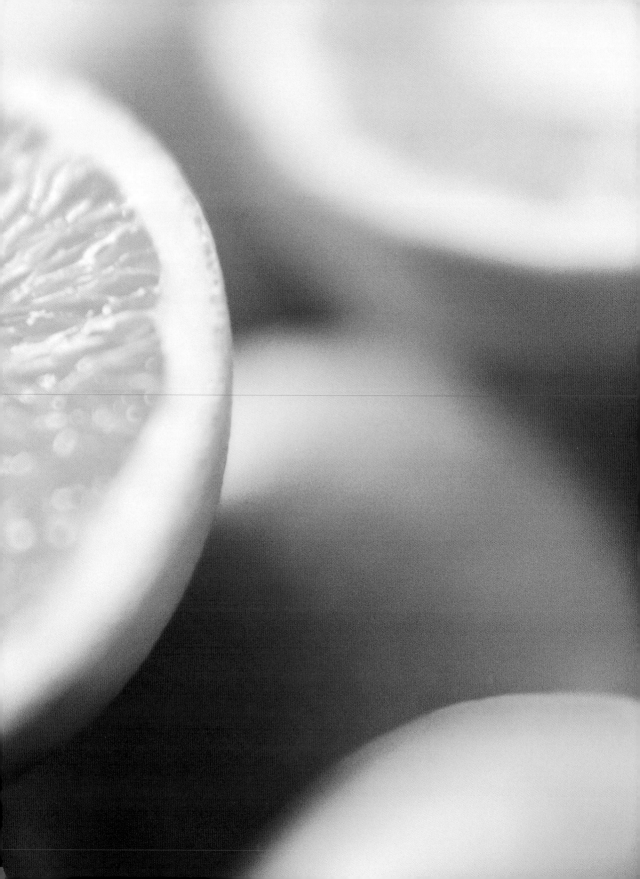

1 HOW THE HOLFORD LOW-GL DIET WORKS

There are five core principles at the heart of the Holford Low-GL Diet. Each of them is a positive guideline in its own right, and each supports the others. All five are easy to follow, and essential if you are serious about achieving permanent weight loss and 100 per cent health:

1 Balance your blood sugar.
2 Eat good fats; avoid bad fats.
3 Eliminate allergies.
4 Supplement for success.
5 Exercise for at least 15 minutes a day.

The 21 days of menus listed on pages 76–81 do all the initial meal planning for you. You can use the recipes as part of your weight-loss diet, or follow the recommendations to modify them for a maintenance diet that will keep you at your ideal weight.

1 BALANCE YOUR BLOOD SUGAR

Keeping your blood sugar balanced is the concept at the heart of the low-GL Diet. As explained in the Introduction, once your blood sugar levels are in balance, sustainable weight loss and 100 per cent health will follow. Success is inevitable.

Keeping your blood sugar balanced depends not only on what you eat, but also on *how* and *when* you eat. Pages 48–49 explain exactly which foods and food combinations stabilise your blood sugar best and help to burn fat. You may be amazed by some of the foods that have a high-GL score, but with understanding of *why* you gain weight (see page 13), comes the ability to control *what* you eat.

In time 'GL-awareness' will become second nature; and before you know it you'll be experimenting by mixing and matching your own combinations of low-GL foods at every meal.

Avoid refined carbohydrates

There are two types of carbohydrate: unrefined and refined. The unrefined carbohydrates are better for you because they are turned into glucose slowly, and your body has more time to use the energy. They tend to be brown in colour: brown basmati rice (which has the lowest GL of all rice), whole grains, brown bread and pasta.

Refined carbohydrates have had all the fibre removed and are to be avoided because they turn into glucose faster than your body can burn it off. They tend to be white in colour: white bread, rice and pasta. Eating too many refined carbohydrates increases your blood sugar levels fast, which produces excess glucose, which turns into fat.

2 EAT GOOD FATS, AVOID BAD FATS

Some fats are essential to health, which is why we have an instinct to eat fat. The body's 'fat sensors' are in your mouth – and we are instinctively drawn towards the creamy texture of fats, sauces, cheese and cream. That's why fat-free diets are such a struggle for most of us. There are 'good' and 'bad' fats in food. Only when you eat the right kind of 'good' fats will your body stop craving that smooth, creamy texture.

I'm 57 years old, 5ft 6in (1.6m) and weighed 16 stone (102kg) last November. I was frightened to death at the rate I was gaining weight. I felt weary and demotivated. I followed your diet and did more exercise ... Now I am maintaining it relatively easily. I feel loads better – more energy, more stamina, more creativity. I feel like I used to feel ten years ago.
Weight Loss: 42lb (19kg) in nine weeks **AD**

GOOD FATS

The 'good fats' are *essential fats* (listed on packets as polyunsaturates) found in seeds, grains and oily fish. They include the essential fatty acids (EFAs) such as omega-3 and omega-6. These fats are essential to health and can help you lose weight. There are two reasons for this. Firstly, your body actually craves essential fats. Secondly, they help your metabolism to work properly: they improve the effectiveness of the brain and the nervous system, they boost immunity, balance hormones and create healthy skin.

Your body and brain depend on omega-3 and omega-6 essential fats. One-quarter of your brain is made up of omega-3s and a lack of essential fats can lead to: lower IQ, poor memory and a tendency to depression. Your hormone balance changes, possibly leading to mood swings, PMS, sugar cravings and weight gain. Your skin dries, and your heart and arteries suffer. This is why these fats are called essential.

Omega-3s carry a host of healthy benefits, not least of which is their ability to boost fatburning:

→ They reduce the risk of heart disease and sudden heart attack.
→ They halve your risk of ever suffering from Alzheimer's disease.
→ They clear up dry skin, stimulate your metabolism, boost brain function, protect your heart and strengthen your immune system.

The low-GL diet gives you exactly the right kind and amount of essential fats, not only to help you stay healthy but also to reduce your desire to eat unhealthy fatty foods.

The Low-GL Diet Made Easy encourages you to:

→ Eat foods high in the essential omega-3 and omega-6 fats, with an emphasis on omega-3 fats from fish, flax and pumpkin seeds, and their oils.
→ Avoid foods high in saturated, hydrogenated or processed fats.
→ Avoid fried, burned or browned food.

Good food sources
Below you'll see the common food sources of these different kinds of fats.

Fat family	Good dietary sources
Omega-3 family	Fish, especially salmon, mackerel, herring, tuna and sardines; flax seeds, pumpkin seeds and walnuts, and their oils.
Omega-6 family	Sunflower, sesame and pumpkin seeds and their oils; also safflower oil, corn oil and soya oil.
Omega-9 family	Olive oil, almonds, walnuts.
Saturated fat	Chicken or turkey, milk, yogurt, eggs (ideally those enriched with omega-3 fats).

BAD FATS
The 'bad fats' are *non-essential* fats (listed on packets as saturated fats, trans-fats and hydrogenated fats) found in meat, dairy products, processed, fried and junk foods. Eating bad fats leaves you unsatisfied, so you'll find yourself craving more fats because your body hasn't received the good fats it needs.

Bad fats feature heavily in the average Western diet and are bad news for your heart, your weight and your arteries. They contribute to diseases such as cancer, diabetes and coronary heart disease, as well as heavy weight gain. If you eat these fats and don't burn them off immediately, all your body can do is store them as unhealthy fat.

Worst of all are the trans-fats and hydrogenated fats. These are the real 'uglies' that have been processed, fried or damaged. When the molecules of essential fats are altered by food processing or frying, they set up a reaction in the body that can damage body cells. That is why some crisps, biscuits, ready-meals and fried foods are bad for you.

There is also an 'in-between' fat (mono-unsaturated): omega-9. Olive oil is a particularly rich source. Whereas this is nowhere near as good for you as the essential 'good' fats, neither is it as bad for you as the non-essential 'bad' fats.

On the Holford Low-GL Diet less than a third of the fat you eat is saturated, compared with two-thirds on the average Western diet.

Foods to enjoy

The omega-3 essential fats, found in flax and pumpkin seeds, and oily coldwater fish such as mackerel, herring, salmon and tuna, keep extra weight at bay in a number of ways. They help make hormone-like substances called prostaglandins, which help to control metabolism and fatburning. They also help to limit the potential damage to the arteries caused when eating too many bad fats or sugary foods leads to bursts of high glucose in the blood.

The omega-6 essential fats, found in hot-climate seeds such as sunflower and sesame, have similar benefits to the omega-3s, and are especially good for the skin and maintaining hormone balance, for example in combating PMS.

Foods to avoid

Foods rich in 'bad' fats include: French fries, hamburgers, deep-fried burgers or nuggets, confectionery, chocolate bars, potato and corn chips/crisps, biscuits, doughnuts, margarine, mayonnaise and most salad dressings.

Unfortunately, many vegetarian processed foods are also high in these hydrogenated fats. Check the label. If it states 'hydrogenated vegetable oils', don't buy it.

In the past, I have tried just about every diet I have ever heard of, even when I knew it wasn't particularly good for me ... Within four days of starting the Holford Low-GL Diet I felt much clearer and more alert, without the fuzziness that I'd lived with for years ... By the second week I was sleeping much better. I'm more optimistic, my mood is better and my energy is loads better. I've lost 12lb (5.5kg) in the first four weeks, and as a result of this success, I have the motivation to change my eating for good ... On the Holford Low-GL Diet, I am rarely hungry and have no desire to give up, which is what has happened in the past. Weight Loss: 12lb (5.5kg) in 4 weeks **DA**

3 ELIMINATE ALLERGIES

Weight gain is a common reaction to foods we're intolerant to. Most of us have intolerances or allergies to certain foods, but few of us are aware of it. Eliminating the food that you are unknowingly allergic to can lead to highly dramatic weight loss.

Water retention, bloating and puffiness are all common allergic reactions, and they make you feel and look fatter. Once you've singled out and eliminated the foods that are triggering your allergic response, you are likely to see dramatic changes very fast. It's not unusual to lose up to 7lb (3.2kg) within three or four days.

Food allergies also cause other problems, such as aches and pains, headaches, fatigue, mood swings and annoying skin and digestive conditions. These also go when you identify and avoid what you are allergic to.

See page 40 for a list of the ten foods that people are most often allergic to. The good news is you can often 'unlearn' your intolerances in as little as three months, which means you can reintroduce previously problematic foods into your diet. If you think you are food sensitive or allergic, it is best to have a proper quantitative IgG ELISA test (see Further Resources, page 155 for more information).

4 SUPPLEMENT FOR SUCCESS

Modern growing methods and long-term storage techniques reduce the nutritional content of foods and there is no guarantee that you are getting all the vitamins and minerals you need from a well-balanced diet, so it is valuable to supplement your diet with additional vitamins and minerals.

There are some 30 vitamins and minerals that are essential for health. Many of them, together with vitamin C, will help you burn fat. They boost your metabolism and reprogramme your body to turn food into energy rather than fat. These aren't drugs, they're nutrients, and they will help fine-tune your metabolism as an integral part of my low-GL weight-loss diet.

FATBURNING SUPPLEMENTS – THE BASICS

I recommend that you supplement your well-balanced diet with fatburning vitamins and minerals to ensure your metabolism is working at peak efficiency. The chart on page 152 gives ideal supplement levels for an average person who is eating a healthful, balanced diet. The easiest way to take these every day is a high-strength multivitamin and mineral, and a 1,000mg vitamin C.

Most health-food shops can help you find supplements to meet these levels in the simplest and least expensive way, choosing from a variety of good brands. Supplements should be taken with food, preferably with breakfast, or spread throughout the day.

FATBURNING SUPPLEMENTS – PULLING OUT THE STOPS

To stabilise your appetite and sugar cravings in the first three months of starting the low-GL diet, I recommend taking, in addition to the vitamin C and multivitamin, a combination of the supplements HCA (hydroxycitric acid), 5-HTP (5-hydroxytryptophan) and chromium. These are the daily levels you need *for the first three months only* especially if you are prone to sugar cravings and have poor appetite control:

⇢ **Hydroxycitric acid (HCA)** works best before meals. One 450mg tablet or capsule twice daily, 30 minutes before lunch and your evening meal.

⇢ **5-hydroxytryptophan (5-HTP)** 50mg taken with carbohydrate (such as fruit) twice daily, with your mid-morning and afternoon snacks. It also gives your mood a boost, but don't take it if you are already taking an anti-depressant.

⇢ **Chromium 200mcg** taken twice daily, with your mid-morning and afternoon snacks.

Supplement facts

If you want the best weight-loss results possible, supplements should not be seen as an optional extra but as a central part of your weight loss and health success. Proper scientific studies show that:

→ Following the Holford Low-GL Diet on its own will enable you to lose weight.

→ Following the Holford Low-GL Diet *and* taking a multivitamin and mineral with vitamin C will help you to lose more weight than the diet alone.

→ Following the diet *and* taking the multivitamin and mineral with vitamin C *and* taking additional chromium, HCA and 5-HTP supplements will lead to *maximum weight loss*.

This means that supplements make a positive and healthy difference to weight loss.

5 EXERCISE – FOR AT LEAST 15 MINUTES A DAY

Exercise – for at least 15 minutes a day – helps to stabilise your blood sugar levels and reduce your appetite.

It seems that the less we move, the more we eat – and vice versa. The human body needs physical activity to work properly, just as it needs water or vitamins. The right kind of exercise will increase muscle and boost the rate at which you burn fat for up to 15 hours afterwards. A pound of muscle burns many more calories a day than a pound of fat, so every pound of fat you lose, and every pound of muscle you gain will further increase your body's long-term ability to burn fat.

To kick-start this process, start by doing 15 minutes exercise a day, or 20 minutes five times a week, or 35 minutes three times a week. Go for it! The short and long-term benefits will far outweigh the initial strain.

KEEP CRAVINGS AWAY ON 40 Ⓖ A DAY

The Holford Low-GL Diet divides the carbohydrate content of foods into low, medium and high. My advice is to eat mainly low-GL foods and food combinations, with occasional medium-GL foods. All in all, that's certainly the fastest way to lose weight and gain energy. High-GL foods (such as sugary snacks) are probably more frustrating than they're worth because eating them simply uses up your daily food allowance, while sending your blood sugar into a spin and increasing your fat reserves.

The limit for each day is 40Ⓖ, because that's the maximum possible for effective and healthy fatburning. You are allowed 10Ⓖ per meal and 5Ⓖ per snack (plus 5Ⓖ for drinks or a dessert):

Breakfast	10Ⓖ
Mid-morning snack	5Ⓖ
Lunch	10Ⓖ
Mid-afternoon snack	5Ⓖ
Evening meal	10Ⓖ
Total	**40Ⓖ**

(Plus 5Ⓖ for drinks or a dessert.)

As long as you don't exceed 40Ⓖ a day you can eat anything. However, eating much more of the best low-GL foods will ensure that you won't go hungry. Either way, you lose weight.

⇢ The low-GL diet reduces your appetite because it stabilises your blood sugar levels so you don't get hungry.
⇢ Sugar cravings take no more than seven days to cure. After that, you'll find that your food cravings will virtually vanish.

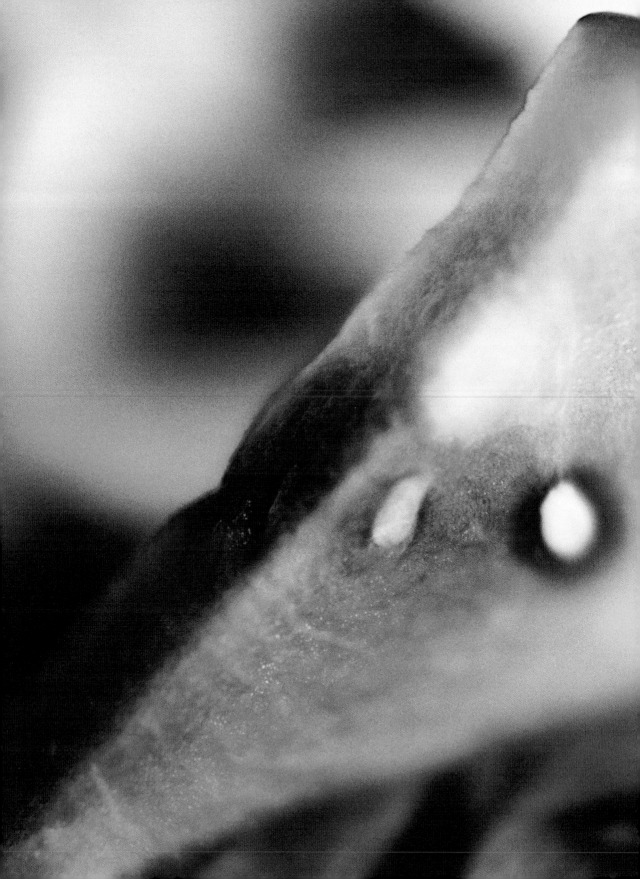

2 THE HOLFORD LOW-GL DIET AND YOU

Each of us is unique, with different health issues and levels of motivation. Starting the Holford Low-GL Diet is like embarking on a personal journey to good health, so it can be helpful to take stock of your state of health before you begin, so that you can see clearly how well you are improving over the next three weeks.

INCREASED ENERGY STARTS HERE

If your blood sugar is out of balance or you have a history of eating 'bad fats' and drinking caffeine-loaded drinks, you probably suffer from low energy levels. From the moment you start following my low-GL diet you will become more alert and able to get through the day without any slump in energy levels and no sense of exhaustion. This is the effect of cutting right back on stimulants and sugar, and supplementing nutrients known to boost energy.

Take the energy test. Are you:

1 More than 7lb (3kg) over your ideal weight?
2 Tired most of the time?
3 Often feeling anxious or stressed?
4 Prone to indigestion or bloating after eating?
5 Suffering from poor memory and concentration?
6 Quite often low or depressed?
7 Plagued by dry skin?
8 Often constipated?
9 Suffering from dark circles or bags under your eyes?

Most people living a Western lifestyle will say 'yes' to an average of seven of these questions. Each is a symptom of being overweight and undernourished – and the reality is no joke. By following the low-GL guidelines, you can be completely free of these symptoms, as well losing 6lb (2–7kg) or more within the next 21 days.

YOUR RELATIONSHIP WITH FOOD

Lasting weight-loss success is related partly to your understanding of food and what it does to your body, and partly to your mind and how you think. What kind of relationship do you have with food? Do you live to eat, or eat to live? Are you able to control your diet quite easily, or does food rule your life? Whether you are interested in low-GL as a way to improve your health, lose weight effectively, or both, my Holford Low-GL Diet will help you to listen to your body and to learn the difference between your true hunger signals and your cravings. Importantly, it will also reintroduce you to the taste and flavour of food.

Eating is essential for life and we crave food from the moment we are born. For most, the early months of feeding are connected to feelings of comfort and safety. However, as we get older, the message becomes more mixed. By the time we reach adolescence, most girls will associate being attractive with being thin, and most boys will have been told to 'eat up, if you want to become big and strong'. Sweets are usually given as rewards (or withheld as punishment) and are associated with pleasure and comfort. Ask yourself the following questions:

⇢ Do you reach for chocolate or other high-fat foods when you are upset?
⇢ Do you gain or lose weight when you are in love?
⇢ Do you reward or punish yourself with food?
⇢ Do you feel the need always to finish what is on your plate?
⇢ Do you eat and drink more when you are out with friends?
⇢ Do you eat more or less when you are under pressure?

A 'yes' to any of these questions means your emotions rather than your appetite sometimes drive your eating. In some people this can lead to eating disorders, compulsive and obsessive eating, and crash dieting. Healthy eating encourages healthy thinking. The following keys to positive thinking will help you to understand your relationship with food:

Self-awareness Understanding how, why and when: *how* you feel about food and weight-gain, *why* you feel guilty about certain eating habits and *when* food or eating is a problem for you.
Self-acceptance *Appreciation* of who you are, and *acceptance* of your needs, your wants and your problems.
Personal action A *commitment to change*. Choose just one situation where eating (or not eating) becomes your comfort trigger. Now think of an alternative, non-food way of coping with the situation. Write that down as your personal target for the week. By stopping each negative habit for a week you will see that you can *choose* your response to your emotions.

How you cope with your emotions does not have to involve food. That is why on the Holford Low-GL Diet you will not find sugary snacks and desserts associated with 'treats'. I believe in other ways to pamper yourself that are more enjoyable (such as treating yourself to a massage, new clothing, a haircut, or a night out with friends). High energy levels and 100 per cent health are the real benefits of balanced eating. The low-GL diet will help to keep you on track by banishing food cravings.

Convenience foods and eating 'on the run' mean it is easier than ever before to reach for unhealthy food, or to overeat. Take a look at the following scenarios and the low-GL way to keep out of trouble and keep your blood sugar on track.

Choose just one action point to change this week. Make a commitment to change one behaviour per week. You will see improvement in no time.

	Unhealthy behaviour	Low-GL answer	Healthy behaviour
Portion sizes	You take your cue for when to stop eating from the size of the packet or the portion.	Get in the habit of leaving some food on your plate (or in the packet) and storing it for tomorrow	You can leave half a packet of crisps, a half-eaten chocolate bar, or some of your lunch without craving or guilt.
Snacking	If you have access to snacks you will keep eating all day.	Pre-prepare healthy snacks such as fruit, raw vegetables, hummus, nuts and seeds.	You don't buy unhealthy snacks, and know when you feel hungry.
Eating out	You find it hard to say 'no' to what's on offer and feel too embarrassed to turn down the sweet dessert.	Plan ahead and decide to choose olives rather than bread, more vegetables rather than protein. Don't feel that you have to eat dessert (or to finish off your portion).	You tell your host in advance that you may eat only a small portion, but if you do eat a little too much you don't worry: you just start again the next day.
Convenience food	Convenience food, and fast and processed foods are easy and cheap, and so remain tempting.	The long-term cost to health is expensive. Remind yourself that this kind of food is heavy in additives, salt and sugar, and low in nutrients.	You decide that your health is important enough to give up convenience food for good.
Emotional eating	You feel guilty that you have lost control.	Don't beat yourself up or feel guilty, as you will be no further forward. Talk to yourself kindly and with respect. Keep a food diary.	You ask yourself what triggered the behaviour and try to deal with it.

This material has been adapted from a handout used by the Patrick Holford Zest4life clubs. See www.holforddiet.com for further information.

BODY FAT AND YOUR IDEAL WEIGHT

All diets focus on weight loss, and there is general acceptance that the closer you are to your ideal weight, the healthier you will be, with less risk of life-threatening and debilitating diseases. However, your weight is only a part of the picture. Your lean muscle tissue is important as well. Vital body organs, such as your heart, liver and kidneys, need to be supported by lean tissue, as does your whole body. That is why fitness is so important. When we exercise we shape up on the inside as well as the outside.

Muscle uses up more glucose, and therefore calories, than fat meaning that muscle (or lean mass) helps you burn fat. This means that if you are heavy, but fit, your weight may not be as much of a problem as you think. On the other hand, if you are thin, but lightweight and lacking in muscle tone, you may not be as fit as you suppose. How can this be?

The reason is, your body is made of both fat tissue and lean tissue (made up of muscle and organs). Having much more fat than lean tissue is a health risk. That is why your body-fat percentage is actually more important than overall weight.

The ideal percentage of body fat for a man is no more than 15 per cent.
The ideal percentage of body fat for a woman is no more than 22 per cent.

Yet the average man on a Western diet has a body-fat percentage of over 20, and the average woman's is above 30.

Your body-fat percentage is easily determined using a set of special scales – your local gym should have some, or you can purchase your own set (see Resources section). Alternatively, ask your doctor to calculate it for you.

ARE YOU FOOD SENSITIVE?

One in three people now has specific food intolerances. These can cause weight to pile on, mainly due to water retention and bloating, and will cause fatigue, too. The body lets go of this excess water when you avoid the foods you are intolerant to. If you'd like to read up on allergies in more depth, see *The Low-GL Diet Bible*. (See also page 30.)

The most common allergy-provoking foods are:

- ⇢ cow's milk
- ⇢ yeast
- ⇢ wheat
- ⇢ gliadin grains (in gluten)
- ⇢ oats
- ⇢ eggs
- ⇢ beans
- ⇢ nuts
- ⇢ shellfish
- ⇢ white fish

The cook's notes for each low-GL recipe contained in this book take allergies into account and suggest ways to modify your meals.

HOW STIMULANTS CAN KEEP YOU FAT

One of the hardest – but best – things about the low-GL Diet was the insistence on giving up coffee and stimulants. I had caffeine-withdrawal headaches for the first few days, but began to feel wonderful after that – alert and fit, and thoroughly detoxified. Weight Loss: 10lb (4.5kg) in four weeks **C**

Do you reach for a cup of tea or coffee routinely throughout the day? Do you think of yourself as a chocoholic? Or are you having trouble kicking the cigarette habit? If you answer yes to one or more of these questions, then stimulants may be making you fat. When you start the day with a caffeine kick or find sugary snacks irresistible, you upset your blood sugar levels and release too much of the stress hormone, adrenaline, into your body.

If you are a smoker you won't need me to tell you that cigarettes destroy many nutrients, but you may not know that smoking also contributes to being overweight. If you can choose to stop smoking – one day at a time – the benefits will be immense and immediate. Your doctor will be pleased to provide support if you ask.

Caffeine (in chocolate, coffee, tea, colas and energy drinks) and nicotine trigger the brain's 'feel-good' chemicals (including dopamine and adrenaline). These chemicals break down stores of sugar held in your body and raise your blood sugar level very quickly, which has the same effect as eating high-GL foods. As your body craves more of the stimulant, so the swings in your blood sugar levels become harder to control. These lead to fatigue, mood swings, anxiety, sugar craving, weight gain and further dependence. The simple answer is to give up all stimulants. But don't do it all at once. Plan to quit, but begin the diet first. This will help to stabilise your blood sugar levels, which will reduce your cravings. You'll then find it easier to give up the stimulants.

THE WONDER OF WATER

We could not function without water. It helps detoxify the body effectively and is essential for all your body's vital organs to work well. Water is also one of the secrets of having healthy skin.

However, the body does not always store water in the right place. If you suffer from unexplained puffiness or bloating, especially on your arms, around the eyes, on your abdomen, or if your fingers or ankles swell, you may be suffering from water retention. Other common signs are dry skin, dandruff, sudden fluctuations in weight, breast tenderness and a tendency towards allergies.

How can you have dry skin and yet have water retention? The answer lies in your body's fats. Your body is made up of two-thirds water and your body cells have a membrane made of special essential fats that keeps the right amount of water in, and outside your cells. These 'good' fats help eliminate water in the wrong places, as well as rehydrating the skin.

The main reasons for water retention are:

⇢ A lack of essential fats.
⇢ Too much sugar in the body.
⇢ Too much salt in the body.
⇢ Allergic reactions to food.

To overcome water retention you need to follow the five principles of the low-GL diet (see page 25) and to make sure you are taking supplements rich in omega-3s and omega-6s. In addition:

⇢ Don't add salt to your food.
⇢ Choose 'low sodium' processed foods.
⇢ Drink eight glasses of water a day (including herb teas).
⇢ Have an allergy test to identify your trigger foods.

Special note
The first 4lb (1.8kg) of weight lost on a high protein, low-carbohydrate diet is more likely to be related to water loss than fat. The weight will return. (See page 83.)

SETTING GOALS TO HELP SUCCESS

The key to low-GL diet success is goal setting and planning ahead. Setting and reviewing daily targets will help you to achieve your goal *step by step*. Instead of saying 'I *wish* I could' or 'I *hope* I can' lose weight, start saying 'I *will* lose weight' while making clear plans based on the diet principles to achieve your goal.

Most people start diets hoping that the weight they have gained over several months or years will disappear in a fortnight, but this is unrealistic (and would also be unhealthy). The purpose of the Holford Low-GL Diet is to *reprogramme* your body to burn fat. As well as helping you to lose weight, the diet will change your body's chemistry. This takes around 20 days. Once past the 20-day mark you will not only be feeling amazing but also your body will have become far more efficient at burning fat.

⇢ **Be realistic** Set yourself targets for changing your diet and taking exercise that you know you will reach.
⇢ **Be patient** Take things one step at a time. It is very hard for the body to lose more than 2lb (1kg) of actual fat in a week. Anything more rapid is likely to be mainly the short-term loss of fluid.

SETTING TARGETS
Generally speaking, a good target to aim for during the first 21 days is to lose 4–6lb (2–3kg) – that's 2lb (1kg) per week. This is easily achievable on the Holford Low-GL Diet. To help decide your target weight, ask yourself:

1 What weight would you like to be, ideally? (The chart on page 153 shows your ideal weight range for your height.) Please make sure your target is within this range.
2 What do you weigh now?
3 What, in your opinion, is your ideal weight?
4 When were you last that weight? (If you are over 40 and wishing you were 18 again, you may need to revise your target!)
5 Is low activity contributing to your weight gain?

Your answers will help you decide your ultimate goal and work out how much exercise you need and how many weeks it will take to achieve your goal based on losing an average of 2lb (1kg) per week.
    The following chapters tell you what to eat and how much to eat, for breakfast, lunch, dinner and snacks.

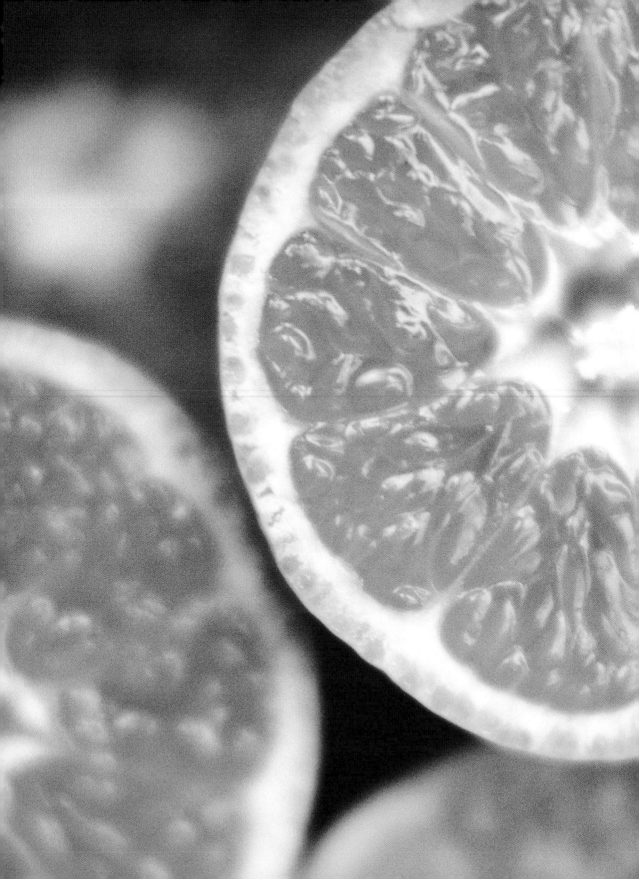

3 LOW-GL WEIGHT-LOSS RULES AND WONDERFOODS

Now that you understand the core principles of low-GL eating and have decided on your personal goals, it is time to take a closer look at what you can eat, and how much you can eat, on the Holford Low-GL Diet. You won't need to worry about rigid discipline, hunger pangs, expensive foods or excluding foods. Just focus on eating low-GL foods and the rest will take care of itself.

There are two main stages to the Holford Low-GL Diet:
Stage one The weight-loss diet will take you to your target weight.
Stage two The maintenance diet is a diet for life.

And there are five main rules for the weight-loss diet:
1 Eat no more than 40🄶🄻 a day (or 55🄶🄻 on the maintenance diet).
2 Have an additional 5🄶🄻 for drinks and desserts (or 10🄶🄻 on the maintenance diet).
3 Practise meal-balancing at every meal.
4 Eat regular snacks.
5 Use the diet on six days out of seven.

Following the guidelines will make sure the weight stays off and that you don't lose too much weight. Achieving this could not be easier. All you need to do is to follow the recipe guidelines in Chapters 6, 7 and 8. To help your body achieve 100 per cent health and to lose weight as effectively as possible, remember also to:

⇢ Choose good fats, avoid bad ones (see page 27).
⇢ Avoid foods that you are allergic or sensitive to (see page 30).
⇢ Take the recommended supplements (see page 31).
⇢ Exercise regularly (see page 32).

YOUR DAILY GL TOTAL

Eat the right ⓖⓛ for your needs. You now know that the GL rating tells you what your food or meal does to your blood sugar, and how it will affect your weight and energy levels. By choosing to eat foods that contain low-GL carbohydrates you will keep your blood sugar in balance and your metabolism functioning effectively, so your body can't help but lose excess weight.

During the weight loss phase of your diet it is important to keep your daily ⓖⓛ to a total of 40 (plus 5ⓖⓛ for drinks and/or desserts). Once you've reached your target weight you need to stabilise and maintain your weight. This is the maintenance phase, when you can increase your overall total by 20 more ⓖⓛ per day. That's an increase of 5ⓖⓛ for breakfast, lunch and dinner plus an extra 5ⓖⓛ for drinks or desserts. You could have a larger portion size of rice, pasta or potatoes in your main meals.

Daily total for weight loss	Daily total for maintenance
10ⓖⓛ for breakfast	15ⓖⓛ for breakfast
+	+
5ⓖⓛ mid-morning snack	5ⓖⓛ mid-morning snack
+	+
10ⓖⓛ for lunch	15ⓖⓛ for lunch
+	+
5ⓖⓛ mid-afternoon snack	5ⓖⓛ mid-afternoon snack
+	+
10ⓖⓛ for dinner	15ⓖⓛ for dinner
(+ 5ⓖⓛ for either a drink or dessert)	(+ 10ⓖⓛ for either drinks or dessert)
Total: 45ⓖⓛ	Total: 65ⓖⓛ

5 **GL** FOR DRINKS AND DESSERTS

You will have extra **GL** for drinks and desserts: either 5**GL** or 10**GL** (see opposite), depending on whether you're on the weight loss or maintenance plan. Desserts are best avoided or limited. They are non-essential, and far from being a 'treat' will often undo all the good you have done over the preceding days as well as limit the quantities of other foods you can eat in a day. Stick to fruit snacks for a natural source of sugar, and look at pages 138–142 for some delicious dessert options.

Water is your key to success. Aim to drink the equivalent of eight glasses of water a day (including non-caffeine herbal teas or diluted juices). A large percentage of so-called hunger pangs is, in fact, thirst.

→ **Coffee alternatives** If you're addicted to cappuccino, try Teeccino, made with a cafetière, or 'instant' chicory drinks with some frothed milk and a touch of cinnamon.
→ **Tea alternatives** If you're addicted to tea, try rooibos (red bush) tea with milk. Herb and fruit teas are also delicious, and widely available.

Low-GL drinks tips
→ Don't exceed more than 5**GL** for drinks and desserts combined.
→ Avoid alcohol for the first two weeks when trying to lose weight in order to kick-start your weight loss.
→ After the first two weeks have no more than 1 unit of alcohol per day (even if this is under 5**GL**!).

Juices

Fruit juices, whether concentrated or fresh, have a relatively high GL because the fibre in the fruits has been removed. They should be diluted before drinking.

The following table shows how much juice equals 5☻ per day:

Tomato juice	600ml (1 pint)
Carrot juice	small glass, about 125ml (4fl oz)
Grapefruit juice, unsweetened	small glass, about 110ml (3³/₄fl oz)
Apple juice, unsweetened	small glass, about 100ml (3¹/₂fl oz), diluted 50/50 with water
Orange juice, unsweetened or the juice of 1 orange	small glass, about 96ml (3¹/₄fl oz), diluted 50/50 with water
Pineapple juice, unsweetened	half a small glass, about 80ml (2¹/₂fl oz), diluted 50/50 with water
Cranberry juice drink	half a small glass, about 80ml (2¹/₂fl oz), diluted 50/50 with water

PRACTISE MEAL-BALANCING

Meal-balancing means eating a combination of both carbohydrate and protein foods at every meal. It is an important concept, at the heart of the low-GL diet. Protein foods (such as fish, eggs, meat and dairy produce), or vegetarian proteins (such as tofu or pulses), have virtually no effect on blood sugar level, and we only need small portions to feel filled up. However, proteins are often high in fat, especially 'bad' fats rather than the omega-3 and omega-6 essential 'good' fats. Eaten on their own and in large quantities they are bad news for our health. However, eating them with low-GL starchy carbohydrates and non-starchy vegetables results in high energy, low blood sugar and optimum health, so you will feel less hungry for longer, lose more weight permanently and supply your body with the essential fats that it needs for good health.

The easiest way to make protein–carb combining a part of your daily life is to keep your food in the following proportions:

⇢ A quarter of each main meal should be protein.
⇢ A quarter of each meal should be carbohydrate: starchy vegetables or other starchy foods.
⇢ Half of each meal should be non-starchy vegetables.

A similar principle applies to snacks. Fiona McDonald Joyce supplies a range of easy suggestions on pages 96–97.

To get an idea of how the low-GL diet tackles hunger, and what it looks like in meal form, first imagine a plate (see below). Now divide it in half. In any main meal, one of those halves can be filled with a selection of the non-starchy vegetables listed below. Now divide the other half in half. One quarter is protein: fish, chicken, lamb or vegetarian proteins such as tofu or beans. The other quarter is a low-GL carbohydrate food serving: bread, potatoes, pasta, starchy vegetables or any other. For guidance on how much of each of these foods equals a portion, see the recipes in Chapter 7 and refer to the tables in Chapter 6.

Main Meals

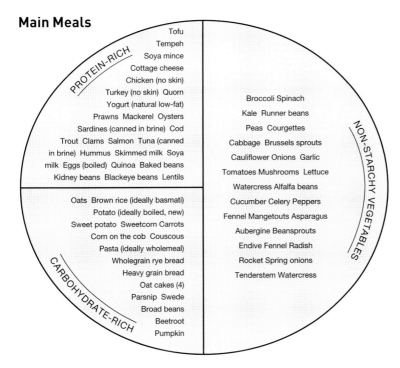

PROTEIN-RICH
Tofu
Tempeh
Soya mince
Cottage cheese
Chicken (no skin)
Turkey (no skin) Quorn
Yogurt (natural low-fat)
Prawns Mackerel Oysters
Sardines (canned in brine) Cod
Trout Clams Salmon Tuna (canned in brine) Hummus Skimmed milk Soya milk Eggs (boiled) Quinoa Baked beans Kidney beans Blackeye beans Lentils

CARBOHYDRATE-RICH
Oats Brown rice (ideally basmati)
Potato (ideally boiled, new)
Sweet potato Sweetcorn Carrots
Corn on the cob Couscous
Pasta (ideally wholemeal)
Wholegrain rye bread
Heavy grain bread
Oat cakes (4)
Parsnip Swede
Broad beans
Beetroot
Pumpkin

NON-STARCHY VEGETABLES
Broccoli Spinach
Kale Runner beans
Peas Courgettes
Cabbage Brussels sprouts
Cauliflower Onions Garlic
Tomatoes Mushrooms Lettuce
Watercress Alfalfa beans
Cucumber Celery Peppers
Fennel Mangetouts Asparagus
Aubergine Beansprouts
Endive Fennel Radish
Rocket Spring onions
Tenderstem Watercress

Foods (and drinks) that are 'out'

→ Avoid sugar in its many disguises and foods that contain fast-releasing carbohydrates with a high-GL score.

→ Avoid bad fats, which occur in foods high in saturated, hydrogenated, processed fats or damaged fats, such as sausages, fried food and junk food.

→ Stop eating any foods you're allergic to, and find alternatives.

→ Avoid alcohol during the first two weeks to a month on your diet, as its effect on the blood is similar to sugar.

→ Limit or avoid caffeinated drinks. Ideally, avoid coffee altogether and have no more than two cups of weak tea a day. Caffeinated fizzy drinks are very bad news as they play havoc with your blood sugar levels and will leave you craving more.

EAT SNACKS

'Graze, don't gorge' is the guideline behind the 'eat snacks' rule. On the low-GL diet, you are trying never to get to the point where your blood sugar drops and you feel ravenously hungry. For that reason 'a little and often' is the norm. By spreading your GLs across the day in line with the guidelines on page 46, you'll avoid energy dips and keep hunger (and cravings) at bay.

THE 'SIX DAYS OUT OF SEVEN' RULE

Few people stick to a diet every single day because life's just not like that. All kinds of challenges intervene, from celebratory drinks to birthday parties and eating out. If you step off track – don't worry about it. My philosophy is that life is to be enjoyed, and food is to be enjoyed. If you feel as if you are in a dieting straitjacket you are more likely to quit altogether. That is why I recommend the 'six days out of seven' rule.

'Six days out of seven' is about personal choice. The rule is that every seventh day you can give yourself 'a day off' – but *only* if you want to. Your choice is to indulge if you want to, or keep to the

40🅖🅛 rule if you want to. Either choice is fine. You will succeed in the long run whichever choice you make. The most important thing to do is to get back on track the next day.

I am not trying to encourage binge eating – and indeed, if you have a history of eating disorder, do be careful how you interpret this guideline. I recommend a maximum of an extra 10🅖🅛 on your 'day off' the diet if you want to limit the 'recovery time' when you come back on track.

Treat yourself, but stay on track
In an experiment, two groups of dieters were given an identical milkshake to drink. One group was told it was high in calories, the other group was told it was low in calories. Each group was then given an unlimited amount of ice cream. Which group do you think ate more? It was the group who had been told the milkshake was high in calories. This shows a common trend amongst dieters, who tend to think, 'Ah well, if I have broken the diet I may as well go the whole hog and indulge myself.' There is no need to damage your health and your progress by taking that approach.

These rules are your building blocks to good health and diet success. You get into the rhythm of your new way of eating very quickly because your body will benefit from it, and it will just make sense.

Foods that are 'in'
→ Low-GL carbohydrates *combined with* protein-rich foods. (Combining carbohydrates such as starchy vegetables, grains and pasta with protein such as meat, fish or pulses lowers their GL rating.)
→ Whole, unprocessed food, high in soluble fibre (such as brown basmati rice, beans, lentils, oats, wholewheat pasta and wholegrain bread).
→ Foods high in essential fats (the 'good' fats: omega-3 and omega-6), such as cold-water fish, seeds and their oils.

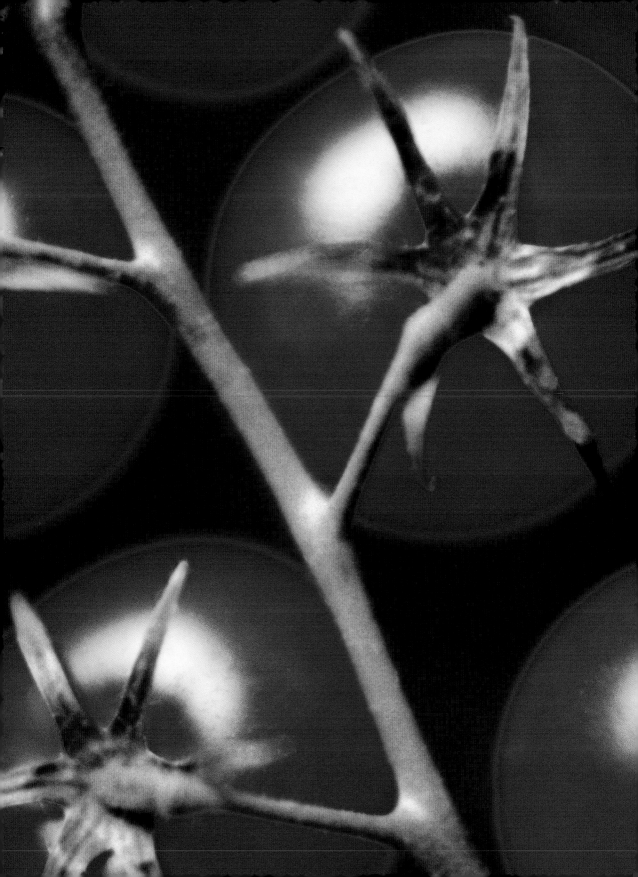

4 THE HOLFORD LOW-GL BODY PLAN

Your body is designed to move, and a certain level of exercise is needed just to keep it working healthily. However, it's all too easy to develop a couch-potato lifestyle, or simply to run out of time to exercise. This is bad news for your long-term health as well as your weight. Low activity levels exaggerate your appetite, slow your rate of metabolism and interfere with your body's ability to keep blood glucose levels stable.

GET THE EXERCISE HABIT

Combining diet and exercise is the best way to lose weight: that way you lose fat, not lean muscle when you diet.

Muscle burns up more energy than fat, so the less muscle you have, the slower your metabolism.

Aerobic exercise (such as brisk walking, jogging, cycling, swimming, dance, skiing, circuit training) increases your heart rate and is ideal for fatburning, whereas anaerobic exercise (using weights or resistance) builds lean muscle and improves body tone. Together they speed up your metabolism and will reduce your body fat percentage. Exercise should be fun as well as healthy, so choose to do something that you enjoy doing, and bring in variety – that way you will hardly notice you are working your body.

'A little and often' is the key to long-term exercise success. Just as healthy weight-loss happens gradually, steadily and permanently, so too the positive benefits of exercise build strongly over time. Yo-yo exercising (occasional bursts of high-intensity exercise) can cause damage to the muscles and ligaments of the body. If you are doing the right kind of exercise, you need spend only 1¼ hours spread over the week to both lose weight and trim your figure. That is just 15 minutes a day (or more if you prefer). What could be easier?

⇢ Write down your goal and set a time span for achieving it.
⇢ Set yourself daily exercise targets: how much will you do and by when.
⇢ Make sure that your goals are realistic and enjoyable.
⇢ Review progress weekly and adjust your goals and outcomes depending on results.

If at first you don't succeed – try something new! But whatever you choose to do, make sure you find something that you will enjoy, and the 15 minutes (or more) will fly by.

WHEN TO EXERCISE

The easiest way to increase your general level of fitness is to get more active all the time. Use the stairs instead of the lift, leave the car at home, and walk or cycle as much as possible. Run around with your kids, take the dog for a walk, take up a sport, or go for a walk instead of watching television.

The best time to do intensive exercise is two hours after eating. If you exercise first thing in the morning, eat a small amount of fruit from your fruit allowance beforehand – and then eat breakfast immediately afterwards. Don't exercise late at night as it will make it much harder for you to sleep. Exercising in natural daylight is ideal because it provides vitamin D via your skin, which means stronger bones.

IT'S NOT ABOUT WEIGHT – IT'S ABOUT FITNESS

During the first four weeks or so of your fitness programme you will lose inches faster than pounds. You'll look trimmer and feel fitter, but the scales may show less weight loss than you had hoped for. Don't be disheartened by what is in fact good news. Muscle is denser and heavier than fat, and so it weighs more. The more lean muscle you gain, the greater your ability to burn fat – and that's what counts. Remember: you are not so much trying to lose weight as aiming to reduce your body fat percentage.

⇢ Choose aerobic types of exercise that raise your heart rate.
⇢ Choose exercise that helps you to build more muscle, which, in turn, burns fat.

BENEFITS OF EXERCISE

Exercise is energising! The benefits are immense. In just two to three weeks you will be enjoying glowing skin, bright eyes and increased vitality.

Drink plenty of water while you're exercising and eat either a balanced snack or a light meal within an hour of finishing a hard workout. Don't let yourself get so hungry that you eat the wrong food. Glucose drinks, energy bars and the like abound, but by now you'll realise that they are not the way to go for fatburning.

Exercise . . .
⇢ Improves digestion
⇢ Improves circulation
⇢ Releases 'feel good' hormones
⇢ Helps relieve stress
⇢ Can improve sleep
⇢ Helps strengthen the heart
⇢ Helps relieve stress
⇢ Improves insulin sensitivity
⇢ Improves muscle tone
⇢ Increases energy levels
⇢ Helps prevent osteoporosis
⇢ Can be sociable and fun.

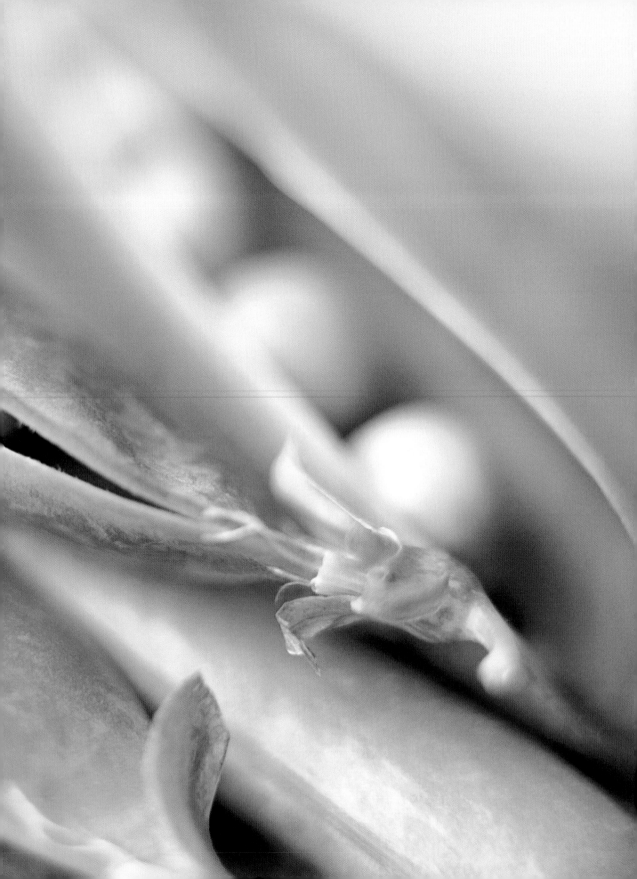

5 GETTING STARTED AND STAYING ON TRACK

Choosing to change your diet and lifestyle doesn't just improve your health, it also changes your life. Even so, it can be a challenge to get started, and hard to stay on track. The keys to success are effective planning – and developing self-belief.

To be successful, you need to plan ahead and set goals, to give yourself time to prepare, both mentally and practically, for your lifestyle change. Deciding in advance what you are going to do and what you want to achieve will build your enthusiasm and help you to commit to the diet, to see off the temptation to stray before you get started.

The most important tip of all is: *Believe you can succeed*. Your self-belief and the way you talk to yourself will influence your ability to stay the course. Supporting each personal 'wish' with a positive programme of action will help you to maintain momentum.

NEVER SKIP BREAKFAST

Whatever you do, don't skip breakfast. Starting the day with your blood sugar levels under control is important for success during the rest of the day. When you first wake up your blood sugar levels are low because it has been several hours since you last ate. Opting for quick energy boosts in the form of sugary snacks, croissants or stimulants, such as tea, coffee, chocolate or cigarettes, will lead to blood sugar lows soon afterwards.

Plan ahead to eat protein with carbohydrate at every meal to slow down the release of sugar. Toast with jam is a bad idea because it is a pure carbohydrate combination, high in sugar and with very high GL. Add protein from eggs instead. The recipe section starting on page 85 offers plenty of fast options for those who are short of time in the mornings.

SNACKS ARE ESSENTIAL

Snacks are vital on the low-GL diet. The old adage of not eating between meals is turned on its head. For the diet to succeed it is essential to keep your blood sugar even, with no peaks or troughs during the day. Eating two 5 GL 'top up' snacks during the day maintains your blood sugar level; that means, for example, you will be able to avoid the temptation of a sugary snack before your evening meal.

Easy ideas for fast and nutritious snacks are given on pages 96–97. Plan to carry a supply of oat cakes and/or seeds with you to avoid eating biscuits, crisps or other unhealthy options.

FOOD ON THE MOVE

If low-GL choices are likely to be a challenge at lunchtime, the situation is best solved by preparing your own food in advance. Make up your salads and snacks, and then store and transport them in storage containers – it is a better value option as well as a healthier one! (Pages 98–115 are rich in delicious ideas.)

Eating out is easy if you plan ahead and decide in advance what you can and can't eat. However, it is a minefield if you leave things to chance. Chapter 8, pages 145–149, provides a rundown of the low-GL options available.

❛ I have had a problem with my weight for 20 years, ever since the birth of my first baby really. Over that time I have been on every diet available, losing some weight unbearably slowly, then putting it back when I could go hungry no longer ... And then I found the Holford Low-GL Diet and lost 22lb (10kg) in two months ... Why did no one ever tell me before? This is not a difficult way to eat, and I don't feel starving hungry at all. My body feels balanced for the first time. Weight Loss: 22lb (10kg) in two months SW ❜

Success tips

→ Write down your goals and the timeframe you have set yourself, and put it in a prominent position where you will notice it and can add progress notes to it every day.

→ Stock up with low-GL foods and drinks in advance (at work as well as at home), so that you can make starting and staying on the diet as easy as possible.

→ Practise healthy cooking methods, as explained on pages 86–88.

→ Make a conscious decision to try new foods. All recipe ingredients are readily available in your local health-food shop, supermarket or a good greengrocer.

→ Remove all high-GL temptations from your fridge and your cupboards. (If your family is likely to be eating in a different way to you, allocate a cupboard or storage area for your foods.)

→ Use the store cupboard guidelines in this chapter to stock up on staple foods and make shopping lists for recipe ingredients rather than leaving things to chance.

STOCK UP WITH ESSENTIALS

Stocking up in advance with essential low-GL foods and getting used to buying and using new ingredients and cooking methods is part of your preparation for 'made easy' success.

Some of the foods listed here may be unfamiliar to you at this point, but exploring new flavours is part of the fun of the low-GL diet. A good supermarket or your local health-food store will stock almost all of the items.

Nothing here is difficult to source or particularly pricey. As always, go for organic wherever possible. Not only is organic produce relatively free of contamination by herbicides and pesticides but it is also good value. The mineral levels in fruit and vegetables can be 100 per cent higher than those of non-organic produce.

Fresh fruits and vegetables

Choose from the following when you go shopping, and where possible, choose foods that are locally grown and in season:

→ Apples, pears, plums, apricots, all berries, oranges, gooseberries, cooking apples, rhubarb, blackcurrants, bananas.
→ Mixed berries, raspberries (frozen).
→ Lemons, unwaxed if possible.
→ Lettuce, rocket, watercress, cherry tomatoes, cucumber, spring onions, alfalfa sprouts, cress, spring onions, beansprouts.
→ Mushrooms, spinach, celery, red and yellow onions, shallots, broccoli, peppers, avocado, parsley, carrots, courgettes, aubergines, peas (fresh or frozen).
→ Baby new potatoes (these have the lowest GL of all potatoes), sweet potatoes.
→ Fresh herbs, such as basil, flat leaf parsley, coriander and chives.
→ Garlic and fresh root ginger.

Foods for your fridge

You don't have to wave goodbye to cheese or butter on the low-GL diet. Fresh fish, tofu and chicken will also be welcome. Try:

→ Skimmed milk or a dairy-free alternative such as soya. (Rice milk, however, has a high GL, so avoid it.)
→ Low-fat cottage cheese and cream cheese, as well as feta, halloumi and soft, mild goat's cheeses.
→ Butter (used occasionally, but keeps for a while).
→ Live natural yogurt, very low-fat.
→ Fresh sardines, cod, haddock, mackerel, herring, salmon.
→ Fresh free range (and organic) chicken.
→ Tofu (soya beancurd) or tempeh (fermented soya beancurd).
→ Anchovies in olive oil (fresh, from the delicatessen counter).
→ Mixed antipasti, preferably in olive oil.
→ Marinated artichoke hearts in oil and canned artichoke hearts.
→ Olives.
→ Unsalted, unroasted nuts and seeds for snacking and cooking. These should be stored in your fridge.
→ Pumpkin seed butter.
→ Organic or free range eggs (ideally enriched with omega-3).

Store-cupboard staples

These staple ingredients will ensure that you are always able to rustle up a low-GL meal at a moment's notice.

- Low-GL Get Up & Go (a delicious smoothie mix that you blend with fruit. See Further Resources, page 155).
- Xylitol (a naturally sweet, low-carb sugar alternative that has 40 per cent fewer calories than sugar).
- Low-sodium salt, or sea salt (to be used in moderation).
- Black peppercorns.
- Marigold Reduced-salt Vegetable Bouillon powder.
- Whole organic rolled oats and oat flakes.
- Wheatgerm.
- Whole barley and rye flakes.
- Cornflour.
- Quinoa ('keen-waa'). This fruit looks and cooks like a grain.
- Dried or canned legumes and pulses. (Canned varieties should be rinsed to remove as much salt and sugar as possible.)
- 100 per cent rye bread – pumpernickel-style or sourdough.
- Rough oatcakes (sugar free).
- Wholemeal pasta.
- Brown basmati rice (this has the lowest GL of all rice so is the only one recommended on the Holford Low-GL Diet).
- Dried herbs and spices.
- Canned tomatoes, tomato purée and sun-dried tomato paste.
- Coconut oil (although it is a saturated fat, it is a very stable oil. It will not raise cholesterol or produce harmful fats when cooked).
- Extra virgin olive oil for salad dressings.
- Sesame oil.
- Mirin, or Japanese rice cooking wine.
- Tamari, a wheat-free soy sauce.
- Tahini (ground sesame seed paste).
- Crunchy peanut butter (choose a sugar-free brand).
- Vanilla and almond extracts.
- Good-quality dark chocolate (around 70 per cent cocoa solids).
- Good-quality anchovies and sardines canned in olive oil.

Now that your kitchen is fully stocked, you're ready to begin. In the next section you'll find useful menus for use on both a weight-loss and maintenance diet.

THE LOW-GL WONDERFOODS

All low-GL foods will help to maintain your blood sugar levels, but there are some that could be considered as 'wonderfoods' for their all-round benefits to nutritional health and well-being. These are the shopping priorities and include the best foods for breakfasts and snacking.

Strawberries, raspberries and blueberries have the lowest GL rating of all fruits. They are delicious on their own or with yogurt, or mixed with other berries, and are packed full of antioxidant vitamins as well.

Tomatoes are great for your waistline, whether fresh and raw, in soups, or in fresh tomato sauces. However, make sure you don't choose the ones with added sugar, such as tomato ketchup. If you drink 600ml (1pint) of tomato juice it has the same effect on your blood sugar as half a glass of a sugared drink – so you get double the benefit as well as lots of nutrients.

Olives are highly nutritious. You can eat them in quantity while maintaining your blood sugar level. Drain first.

Oatcakes manufactured by Nairn's have the lowest GL rating of all those tested. They are delicious alternatives to bread.

Xylitol is a natural sugar, extracted from plants, particularly plums, and has 40% fewer calories than refined sugar, although it tastes just as good.

Low-GL Get Up & Go (1 scoop = 3 ⓖ) is an all-in-one powder which is excellent for digestive and hormonal health, and is full of fibre. It contains a highly nutritious mix of protein, derived from quinoa, soya and rice, plus carbohydrate from organic apple powder. Minerals and essential fats are also in the mix, from almonds and flax seeds to sesame seeds and oat fibre. When mixed with milk and half a banana or berries it becomes an ideal breakfast or snack.

For further information about these and other ingredients, visit my website at www.holforddiet.com.

STAYING ON TRACK

When you're on a weight-loss diet, setting targets is important. Changing your food habits can happen only if you make plans and alter how you think and what you do. In time you will change your behaviour and create a new positive habit.

To illustrate what I mean, a three-week action plan follows, to help plan a new objective each week. Taking small steps that represent consistent progress will take you nearer and nearer your ultimate weight-loss goal.

	Weekly food or drink objective	Weekly activity/exercise objective	Weekly habit objective
Week 1	I will have an alcohol-free week.	I will walk for 10 minutes each morning on the way to work instead of taking the bus.	I will plan this week's meals in advance and write a shopping list.
Week 2	I will try a new food I've never had before (such as quinoa).	I will walk up the escalator instead of standing on it.	I will enjoy a non-food reward. I will take supplements every day.
Week 3	I will drink 6–8 glasses of water/herb tea/caffeine-free tea each day.	I can enjoy 10 minutes of relaxation each evening before starting the evening chores.	I will re-stock my cupboards with low-GL foods. I will ask myself how hungry I am before eating.

YOUR DAILY TARGET

All change and progression has to start where you are, which means keeping a close eye on what you eat and when you eat it.

Think of your daily ⓖⓛ allowance as your GL bank account: the more ⓖⓛ you can 'save' in a day, the more you will be able to use for special treats. But remember, you must keep to 40ⓖⓛ per day for food and 5ⓖⓛ for a drink or dessert; the totals cannot be carried over from one day to the next, nor from one week to the next.

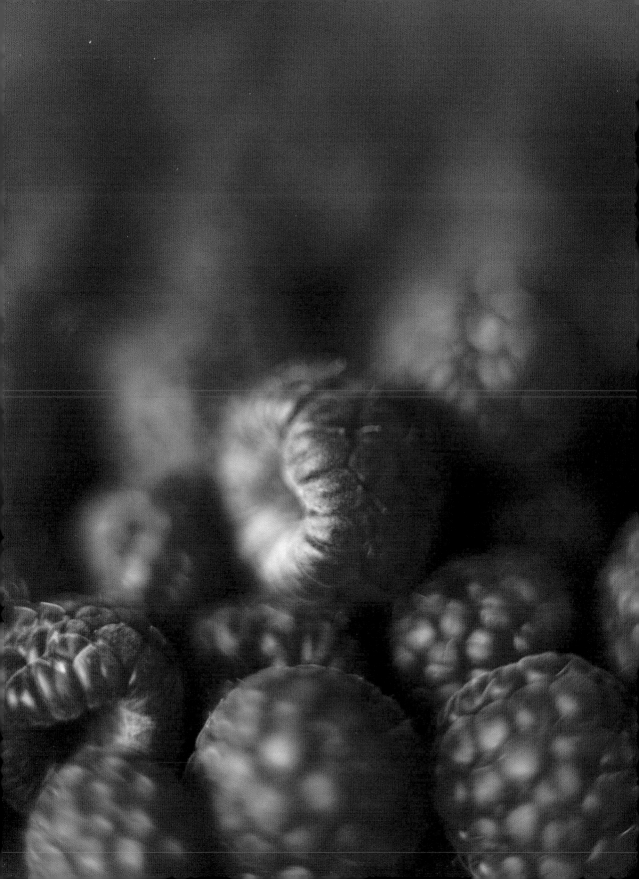

GL CALCULATOR

Below is a blank GL Calculator. You can photocopy this so that you have a new version to carry with you and fill in every day. The GL Calculator helps you keep track of the GLs you consume each day. Simply write down, in the spaces provided, what you have eaten at each meal, and the GL total.

MEAL	DESCRIPTION	TOTAL
Breakfast Aim = 10 GL		
Snack Aim = 5 GL		
Lunch Aim = 10 GL		
Snack Aim = 5 GL		
Supper Aim = 10 GL		
Drinks or puddings Aim = 5 GL		
DAILY TOTAL		

Once you are familiar with the GL values of your favourite foods, change will be easy. However, effective change takes time, and it is important to remember to be patient. Slow and steady is what will get you permanent results. Good luck!

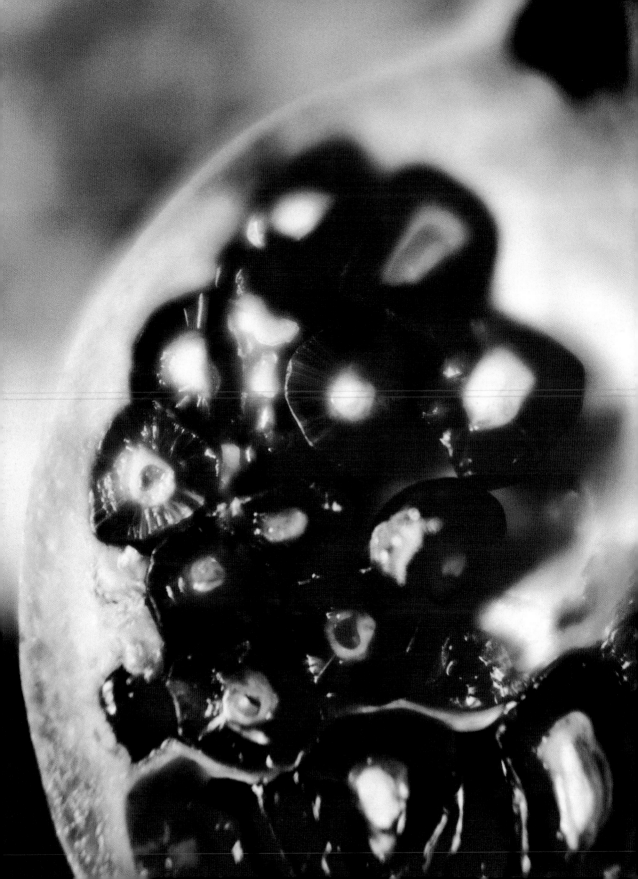

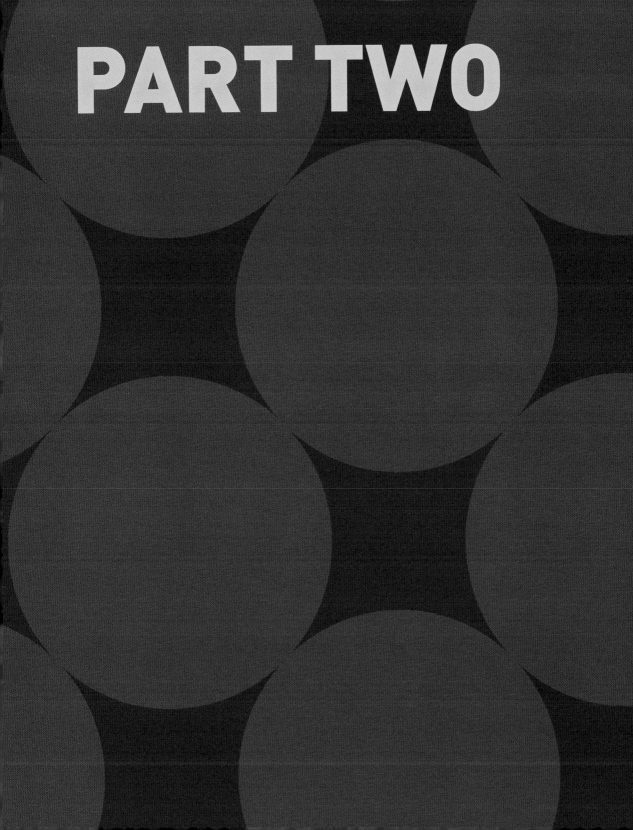

PART TWO

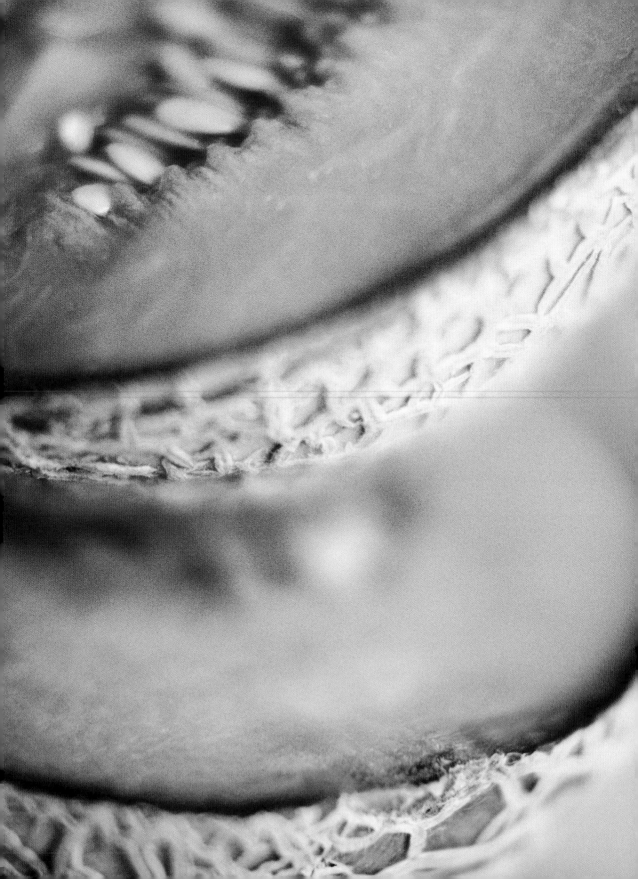

6 THE 21-DAY WEIGHT-LOSS PLAN

The Holford Low-GL Diet is all about freshness, variety, flavour and enjoyment. No foods are banned (although the quantities are limited) and there is scope for infinite variety. Adjusting to your new way of eating couldn't be easier as the first three weeks of the diet are planned out for you day by day. The idea is to give you time to get used to the quantity and balance of foods on the diet. Once you're familiar with the portion sizes and with the basic rules, you can adapt the recipes, create your own, or swap meals from one day to another.

TOP TIPS FOR MENU PLANNING

⇢ Plan ahead so that you know what you are eating for each meal of the day. That way you avoid impulse buying and eating.
⇢ Make sure you are getting the right level of essential fat. Oily fish, for example, occurs in the menus no more than three times a week.
⇢ Stock up on low-GL wonderfoods (page 26) and non-starchy vegetables (page 72) to boost your nutritional wellbeing.
⇢ Ring the changes with your snacks.
⇢ Limit the number of desserts you have each week.
⇢ Keep your menus varied so you don't get bored with any of the ingredients.

Before I started the Holford Low-GL Diet I had almost constant knee pain. In one month this has been all but eliminated, I've lost 5lb (2 kg) in weight, my hair and skin condition has noticeably improved and so has my mood. Weight Loss: 5lb (2kg) in one month TF

TOP TIPS FOR COOKING

→ Buy foods as fresh and unprocessed as possible and eat them soon afterwards.

→ Eat more raw food. Be adventurous. Try raw courgette or beansprouts in salad, for example.

→ Cook foods as whole as possible, slicing or blending before serving.

→ Use as little water as possible, preferably steaming, poaching or steam-frying.

→ Fry foods as infrequently as possible.

→ Favour slow-cooked methods that introduce less heat.

→ Don't overcook, burn or brown food.

→ See more about cooking methods on pages 86–88.

DAILY MEAL ALLOWANCES

The following portion sizes will give you a helpful guide as to how much you should consume as snacks or components of a meal:

HOW BIG IS A PROTEIN SERVING?

The good news is that protein foods have virtually no GL rating because they have low, or no carbohydrate and so do not turn into blood sugar. For optimum health they should be eaten with carbohydrate foods and non-starchy vegetables, and should make up no more than a quarter of your meal. These servings are simply the amount needed to meet most people's protein requirements, but are not necessarily reflective of what you would eat, so you can have more than a quarter of a can of tuna, for example.

Protein	Serving weight	Serving size
Tofu and tempeh	160g (5³/₄oz)	³/₄ packet
Soya mince	100g (3¹/₂oz)	3 tbsp
Chicken (no skin)	50g (1³/₄oz)	1 very small breast fillet
Turkey (no skin)	50g (1³/₄oz)	¹/₂ small breast fillet
Quorn	120g (4¹/₄oz)	¹/₃ pack
Salmon and trout	55g (2oz)	1 very small fillet
Tuna (canned in brine)	50g (1³/₄oz)	¹/₄ can
Sardines (canned in brine)	75g (2³/₄oz)	²/₃ can
Cod	65g (2¹/₄oz)	1 very small fillet
Clams	60g (2¹/₄oz)	¹/₄ can
Prawns	85g (3oz)	6 large prawns
Mackerel	85g (3oz)	1 medium fillet
Oysters		15 oysters
Yogurt (natural, low-fat)	285g (10oz)	¹/₂ large tub
Cottage cheese	120g (4¹/₄oz)	¹/₂ medium tub
Hummus	200g (7oz)	1 small tub
Skimmed milk	440ml (16fl oz)	a little over ³/₄ pint
Soya milk	415ml (15fl oz)	about ³/₄ pint
Eggs (boiled)		2
Quinoa	125g (4¹/₂oz) (dry weight)	1 large serving bowl (cooked weight)
Baked beans	310g (11oz)	³/₄ can
Kidney beans	175g (6oz) (dry weight)	¹/₃ can
Black-eyed beans	175g (6oz) (dry weight)	¹/₃ can
Lentils	165g (5³/₄oz) (dry weight)	¹/₃ can

HOW BIG IS A STARCHY CARBOHYDRATE SERVING?

Your main meal target for starchy carbohydrates is 7ⓒⓑ. These amounts are critical, so take care to weigh before you begin cooking.

Carbohydrate	7ⓒⓑ looks like	Weight, uncooked
Pumpkin/squash	1 serving	185g (6½oz)
Carrot	1 large	160g (5¾oz)
Swede	⅓ swede	150g (5½oz)
Quinoa	2 handfuls	65g (2¼oz)
Beetroot	1 large	110g (3¾oz)
Cornmeal	1 handful (large)	60g (2¼oz)
Pearl barley	1 handful	40g (1½oz)
Wholemeal pasta	1 handful	40g (1½oz)
White pasta	1 handful (small)	35g (1¼oz)
Brown rice	1 handful	35g (1¼oz)
Brown basmati rice	1 handful	40g (1½oz)
White rice	1 handful (small)	25g (1oz)
Couscous	1 handful	25g (1oz)
Broad beans	1 handful (small)	30g (1oz)
Corn on the cob	½ cob	60g (2¼oz)
Boiled potato	1 medium potato	75g (2¾oz)
Baked potato	½ baked potato	60g (2¼oz)
French fries	3 fries	50g (1¾oz)
Sweet potato	½ sweet potato	60g (2¼oz)

HOW BIG IS A NON-STARCHY VEGETABLE SERVING?

Your daily target for non-starchy vegetables is 3ⓒⓑ per day. That's approximately half a dinner plate of steamed vegetables (see page 49). The following can be eaten in almost unlimited quantities because their carbohydrate level is so low:

Asparagus, aubergine, beansprouts, broccoli, Brussels sprouts, cabbage, cauliflower, celery, courgette, cucumber, endive, fennel, garlic, kale, lettuce, mangetouts, mushrooms, onions, peas, peppers, radish, rocket, runner beans, spinach, spring onions, tenderstem, tomatoes, watercress.

HOW BIG IS A FRUIT SERVING?

On the whole you'll be concentrating on low-GL fruit such as plums, berries, pears and watermelon. Aim for two to three servings of fruit every day, for example two as snacks and one with breakfast or in a dessert. You'll notice that you can eat an awful lot of berries for 5 GL – don't worry, this isn't the recommended serving size (as 600g is an awful lot), but it shows you just how low the GL is for these fruits.

Fruit	5 GL looks like	Weight
Blackberries	1 large punnet	600g (1lb 5oz)
Blueberries	1 large punnet	600g (1lb 5oz)
Raspberries	1 large punnet	600g (1lb 5oz)
Strawberries	1 large punnet	600g (1lb 5oz)
Cherries	1 punnet	200g (7oz)
Grapefruit	1 small	200g (7oz)
Pear	1 large pear	150g (5½oz)
Melon (cantaloupe)	½ small melon	150g (5½oz)
Watermelon	1 big slice	150g (5½oz)
Peach	1 peach	120g (4¼oz)
Apricot	4 apricots	120g (4¼oz)
Orange	1 large	120g (4¼oz)
Plum	4 plums	120g (4¼oz)
Apple	1 small	100g (3½oz)
Kiwi fruit	1 kiwi	100g (3½oz)
Pineapple	1 thin slice	85g (3oz)
Grapes	10 grapes	75g (2¾oz)
Mango	1 slice	75g (2¾oz)
Canned fruit cocktail	½ small can	65g (2¼oz)
Papaya, raw	1 slice	60g (2¼oz)
Banana	½ small	50g (1¾oz)
Canned apricots	⅓ small can	50g (1¾oz)
Canned lychees	⅕ x 200g can	35g (1¼oz)
Prunes	3 prunes	30g (1oz)
Dried apricot	3 apricots	30g (1oz)
Dried apple	3 rings	30g (1oz)
Dried figs	1 fig	20g (¾oz)
Sultana	10 sultanas	10g (¼oz)
Raisins	10 raisins	10g (¼oz)
Dates	1 date	5g (⅛oz)

WEIGHT-LOSS MENUS

Following are three weeks' worth of daily menus to get you on the right track towards losing weight. Please note: Day 7 of each week has a bigger lunch and smaller supper. Lunches are taken from the Food on the Move/Working Lunches section of the recipes, and snacks from the 5 GL Snacks section, unless otherwise indicated.

If you find yourself straying back into high-GL or 'bad fat' habits, try focusing on your motives and goals.

⇢ What are *your* links between food, your feelings and behaviour?
⇢ Make a daily plan and put it into action. Once you start to believe in your ability to stay on track, you will trust yourself to go the whole distance.
⇢ Choose one new goal each week. You will gradually replace old unhealthy eating habits with healthy ones.

EASY MEAL SWAPS

Instead of	Have instead
breakfast cereal	porridge
fried egg and bacon	scrambled eggs on rye toast
croissant and jam	fruit salad with yogurt and seeds
burger and chips	sauages with sweet potato mash and onion gravy
spaghetti carbonara	chicken with aubergine and peppers
doner kebab	greek stuffed pitta bread
prawn biriyani	king prawn pilaff
smoked salmon and cream cheese sandwich	smoked salmon with cottage cheese salad
tea, coffee, cola	herb teas, rooibos, fruit juice

HIGH FAT/HIGH SUGAR

The foods listed below are either high in fat or high in sugar, so keep to the recommended amounts per day or week. Many of them have been included in the recipes following.

Food	Guidelines
Dried fruit	choose fresh fruit or dried apricots or prunes (both lower GL)
Coconut	can be used in small amounts to flavour dishes
Seeds	in general, limit to 4 tsp a day, or 1 heaped tbsp
Nuts	same as seeds (although seeds are better)
Salad dressings	stick to the measures given on page 99
Avocados	1 medium avocado, about 190g (6¾oz), twice a week, maximum
Vegetable oil and butter	use sparingly, as in the recipes
Tahini (sesame spread)	use a small amount instead of butter
Fatty fish such as herring, mackerel, tuna, kippers	three times a week, maximum
Chicken (no skin), game	twice a week, maximum
Milk and yogurts	stick to skimmed milk and low-fat yogurt
Eggs	six a week, maximum (ideally omega 3 enriched)

I have over the last two weeks been using your new Holford Low-GL Diet book. I can't believe what a change it has made. I have lost 5lb (2kg) in weight, and 6 inches (from my waistline). Overall I have more energy, don't get so tired, don't feel bloated any more and have lost my sweet-tooth cravings – all in two weeks...I intend to carry on with this. Weight Loss: 5lb (2kg) in two weeks JS

WEEK 1 – GETTING STARTED

Days 1–7 are all about enthusiasm and getting started. Encourage yourself to achieve early successes by keeping strictly to the daily menus. There will be a few ingredients such as quinoa, miso soup and tahini that you may not be used to using every day – but enjoy the experimentation, and give yourself time to get used to new cooking methods and flavours.

DAY 1
Breakfast Porridge
Lunch Chicken, sun-blush tomato and pine nut salad
Dinner King prawn pilaff with steamed vegetables
Snacks Small pot, about 150g (5¹/₂oz) live natural yogurt with berries/2 rough oatcakes with nut butter

DAY 2
Breakfast Fruit salad with yogurt and seeds
Lunch Smoked salmon and cream cheese on rye bread
Dinner Sausage and pepper casserole with boiled baby new potatoes
Snacks Spring onion and radish crudités with 150g (5¹/₂oz) hummus/1 boiled egg with 2 rough oatcakes

DAY 3
Breakfast One-minute muesli
Lunch Hummus and roasted pepper wrap
Dinner Chicken and vegetable steam-fry with brown basmati rice
Snacks Fruit and yogurt smoothie/miso soup and an apple

DAY 4
Breakfast Omelette in pitta bread
Lunch Smoked trout sandwich with tapenade and watercress
Dinner Rice and vegetables with a tahini sauce
Snacks 120g (4¹/₄oz) cottage cheese and 2 plums or crudités/ 2 rough oatcakes with nut butter

DAY 5
Breakfast Breakfast sundae
Lunch Ham, artichoke heart and tomato open sandwich
Dinner Fajitas
Snacks Peach plus 2 tsp sunflower seeds/baby corn and radish crudités with guacamole

DAY 6
Breakfast Toast and nut butter
Lunch Smoked salmon with cottage cheese salad
Dinner Cashew and sesame quinoa
Snacks 2 rough oatcakes with hummus and cucumber slices/handful of olives plus a piece of fruit

DAY 7
Breakfast Scrambled eggs with 1 slice rye toast
Lunch Chicken with aubergine and peppers (see Main Meals)
Dinner Puttanesca pasta with tuna
Snacks Pear plus 2 tsp pumpkin seeds/miso soup plus a handful of olives

Drinks per day Unlimited water, herbal teas and coffee alternatives, plus 1 glass of diluted juice

WEEK 2 – STAYING ON TRACK

Days 8–14 are about staying on track and motivated. So, you've kept your cravings at bay for seven days. That's cause for celebration. Part of the low-GL philosophy is to separate treats from food, so instead of reaching for high-GL snacks or a glass of celebratory wine, why not reward yourself with a different kind of treat? Giving yourself (non-food) treats is very important as it helps you to celebrate and recognise the progress you are making.

DAY 1
Breakfast Breakfast smoothie
Lunch Deli-style pastrami open rye sandwich
Dinner Pesto-baked salmon with boiled baby new potatoes and roasted vegetables
Snacks 1 slice pumpernickel-style rye bread with nut butter/celery and ½ carrot made into crudités with guacamole

DAY 2
Breakfast One-minute muesli
Lunch Mackerel and chickpea salad
Dinner Grilled goat's cheese salad with roasted peppers and walnuts
Snacks Omelette (2 eggs) with 1 slice of toasted pumpernickel-style rye bread/marzipan truffles (see Easy Desserts)

DAY 3
Breakfast Toast and nut butter
Lunch Ham, artichoke heart and tomato open sandwich
Dinner Harissa-spiced tuna steak with quinoa and a mixed salad
Snacks Apple plus 2 tsp Brazil nuts/2 rough oatcakes with cottage cheese

DAY 4
Breakfast Porridge
Lunch Greek stuffed pitta bread
Dinner Sausages with sweet potato mash and onion gravy
Snacks Fruit and yogurt smoothie/pepper and cucumber crudités with hummus

DAY 5
Breakfast Breakfast sundae
Lunch Low-fat egg 'mayo' on oatcakes with salad
Dinner Creamy mushrooms on polenta slices
Snacks Slice of pumpernickel-style rye bread with nut butter and cucumber/pear and 2 tsp almonds

DAY 6
Breakfast Fruit salad with yogurt and seeds
Lunch Greek salad
Dinner Peppers stuffed with smoked mackerel and beans
Snacks Raspberries with sweet tahini sauce (see Easy Desserts)/slice of pumpernickel-style rye bread with cottage cheese and cucumber slices

DAY 7
Breakfast Scrambled eggs and one slice of rye toast
Lunch Pork chops with a mustard and crème fraîche sauce, peas and new potatoes (see Main Meals)
Dinner Chestnut and butterbean soup
Snacks Handful of olives plus a piece of fruit/fruit and yogurt smoothie

Drinks per day Unlimited water, herbal teas and coffee alternatives, plus 1 glass of diluted juice

WEEK 3 AND BEYOND – ACHIEVING YOUR TARGETS

By days 16 to 21 you will begin to feel the benefits of being on the diet. Your skin will have a healthy glow, your clothes will start to fit better and you will be getting used to using ⓖⓛ and portion sizes. Most people by this stage are feeling so good that they are contemplating adopting the low-GL principles for life, not just for three weeks.

DAY 1
Breakfast Breakfast smoothie
Lunch Chicken, sun-blush tomato and pine nut salad
Dinner King prawn pilaff with steamed vegetables
Snacks Apple plus a handful of cashew nuts/2 rough oatcakes with reduced-fat cream cheese

DAY 2
Breakfast One-minute muesli
Lunch Hummus and roasted pepper wrap
Dinner Steamed salmon with stir-fried shiitake mushrooms, brown basmati rice and wilted spinach
Snacks Celery and ½ carrot made into crudités with cottage cheese/2 rough oatcakes spread with tuna and guacamole or salsa

DAY 3
Breakfast Toast and nut butter
Lunch Tuna and tomato salad
Dinner Chicken with aubergine and peppers, with wholemeal pasta and a green salad
Snacks Apple plus 2 tsp sunflower seeds/marzipan truffles (see Easy Desserts)

DAY 4
Breakfast Breakfast smoothie
Lunch Deli-style pastrami open rye sandwich
Dinner Warm tomato and olive mixed-pulse salad with
a green salad
Snacks Slice of pumpernickel-style rye bread with nut
butter/celery and radish crudités with guacamole

DAY 5
Breakfast Porridge
Lunch Goat's cheese, pear and pecan salad
Dinner Hot-smoked fish with a lemon and caper dressing, with
salad and flageolet beans, followed by ten-minute fruit crumble
Snacks Apple plus 2 tsp walnuts/fruit and yogurt smoothie

DAY 6
Breakfast Omelette in pitta bread
Lunch Salade niçoise
Dinner Soya and sesame tofu steam-fry with brown basmati rice
Snacks Pear plus 2 tsp pecan nuts/2 rough oatcakes with nut
butter

DAY 7
Breakfast Fruit salad with yogurt and seeds
Lunch Chicken with cherry tomatoes and crème fraîche
(see Main Meals)
Dinner Chestnut and butterbean soup
Snacks Slice of pumpernickel-style rye bread with
hummus/raspberries with sweet tahini sauce (see Easy Desserts)

Drinks per day Unlimited water, herbal teas and coffee
alternatives, plus 1 glass of diluted juice

WHAT IF THE DIET ISN'T WORKING?

What if you have made it to the end of week three, can see improvements but you are just not losing weight. What has gone wrong?

I can understand how frustrating this must feel. No single diet works for everyone, as there are many different causes of weight gain. The possible reasons below may explain what is holding you back.

Are you losing inches rather than weight?
This is good news. It means that you are making lean muscle, which is heavier, but has the capacity to burn more fat. Keep going. The weight loss will follow.

Are you are still drinking alcohol, sugary drinks and/or caffeine?
If you are and you're not losing weight, it is time to bite the bullet and give them up.

Are you exercising regularly?
Exercise really does help kick-start your metabolism. If your weight isn't shifting, then you need to increase your levels of activity.

Are you taking the supplements?
Supplements do make a difference and, in addition to the basic multivitamin and vitamin C, the combination of chromium, HCA and 5-HTP definitely gives you the edge in appetite control.

Have you had an allergy test?
Don't underestimate the impact of food sensitivity and allergies. Your weight can really get stuck until you remove an offending food. Have a food-intolerance test and avoid your problem foods for a few weeks.

Are your hormones out of balance?
It is possible that you are oestrogen-dominant. Hormonal imbalances can stop you losing weight. You need to get this checked by your doctor, who will advise whether you need to be tested for an underactive thyroid.

I often lose weight fast, but then it all comes back again. What's going on and why can't I lose weight?

The first 4lb (2kg) lost on any diet is inevitably water, not fat. Why do we lose water? It is because the excess sugar from food does not turn straight from glucose into fat. When your glucose level is too high, the body stores it first as glycogen (which is very similar to glucose) and it can be released very rapidly if you're lacking in glucose.

Fat is the long-term store; glycogen is the short-term store.

We all have roughly the same amount of glycogen in our bodies. It is stored mainly in the muscles, with some in the liver – and it is stored with water. When you run out of glucose, because you have reduced your carbohydrate intake, your body starts to break down your glycogen to create more glucose. When this happens you lose all the water it's stored with at the same time – and that's why you lose up to 4lb (2kg) of water on a very low-carb diet. Ultimately, however, your body will replace the missing glycogen – and the water it is stored with – because the body needs it to survive.

⇢ The major cause of obesity is an increase in sugar and refined carbohydrate, not an increase in fat.
⇢ Different sources of calories have different effects on weight loss.
⇢ Eating a low-GL diet triggers more rapid weight loss than any other diet.
⇢ If you eat too few calories your metabolic rate slows down to conserve your fat, so your body sends out an instruction to store more weight.
⇢ High-protein diets stabilise your blood sugar levels and reduce your appetite, but they are nutritionally unbalanced and put too much stress on your liver, so they are not good for you in the long run.
⇢ Low-fat diets are bad for you because the body needs essential fats and keeps craving fats until it gets them. Depriving your body of fat altogether will just increase the craving even more.

I hope that in looking at these solutions you find the one that is likely to work for you. Be patient, be persistent, and good luck.

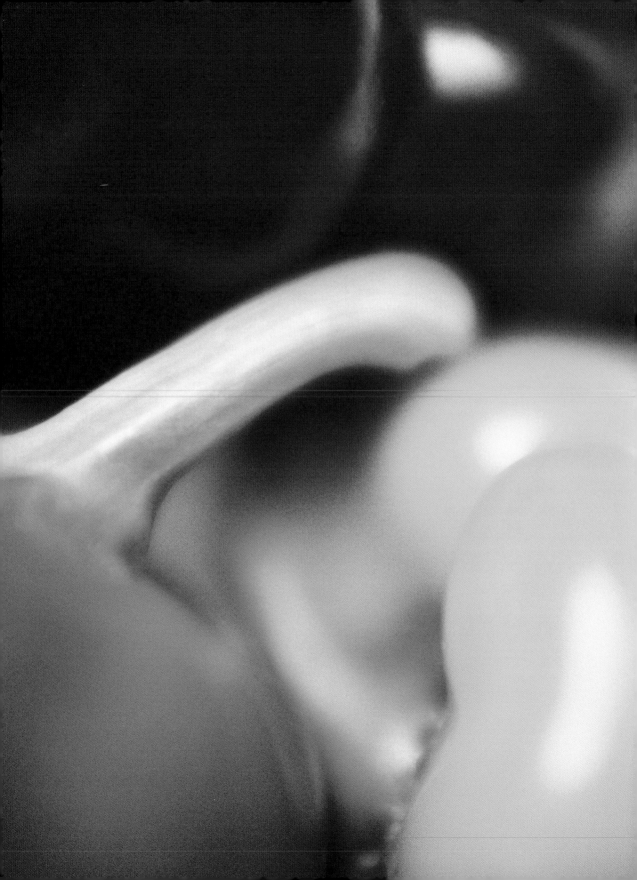

7 RECIPES
FIONA McDONALD JOYCE

The quality and variety of the recipes are all-important when you are losing weight. No matter how reliable the research and no matter how effective the results, unless the food itself is delicious to eat and easy to prepare, it will be hard to stay the course.

Fiona keeps flavour and variety at the centre of her menu planning. All her recipes have been created with busy lifestyles in mind. They feature everyday ingredients and require the minimum of fuss, but do not compromise on flavour, texture, freshness or variety. The recipes are also high in fibre and use ingredients that are naturally high in key vitamins and minerals.

All you need to do is select a breakfast, lunch and dinner for each day, plus two snacks by referring to the menu planners on pages 76–81 or by compiling your own daily menu from the relevant sections in the recipes that follow. Recipes can be modified for vegetarian or special diets, and all can be adapted for use either for the weight-loss or for the maintenance diet. Maintenance portion details are provided at the bottom of each recipe. Look at the Cook's Notes for suggested variations too.

The Holford Low-GL Diet is based mainly on fresh vegetables, fruits, beans, lentils and wholegrains, with some fish and chicken, so you will find it very economical. Budget and availability allowing, I encourage you to buy the freshest ingredients possible, preferably organic, since they are high in nutrients and chemical-free. Vary your choice of fruits and vegetables in line with the season.

Almost all the recipes are sugar-free, using the natural sweetness present in food, or xylitol, a natural plant sugar that has all the taste of sugar but a fraction of the calories. It does not disrupt your blood sugar and has a very low-GL. It is also good for your teeth.

I also suggest seasoning with herbs and with Solo, a special kind of sea salt with little sodium, and loads of health-promoting magnesium and potassium (see Further Resources).

FAT-FRIENDLY COOKING METHODS

Keeping your ⊕ low and your blood sugar level stable depends not only on what you eat but also on how you cook what you eat. Cooking encourages the carbohydrate in foods to be released faster. The longer you cook something and the higher the temperature, the faster the carbohydrate in the food is released. The best method is actually leaving the food raw, but steaming, boiling, poaching, steam-frying, waterless cooking, baking and grilling are all good, too, in that order. Avoid frying food as much as possible. Deep-fried foods are definitely to be avoided.

Steaming

The best way to cook green, leafy, less-starchy vegetables is to steam them, as this will preserve a lot of their vitamins, as well as enhance their flavour. The method can be used for most food, especially fish, but is less successful for starchy vegetables such as potatoes and parsnips, and is not ideal for red meat.

Boiling

Boiling raises the GL of foods more than steaming, but less than baking. To keep the food nutritious and low GL, use very little water, keep the lid on, and cook the food whole if possible, and for as short a period of time as possible. Eat all vegetables (except for potatoes) al dente, that is a little crisp, but not soft.

Poaching

To poach, cover food in liquid, such as water, milk or a flavoured broth, and simmer it gently in the liquid. Poaching is an ideal way to infuse flavour into food.

Steam-frying

As well as giving food a great taste, steam-frying is good for health. The lower temperature used in steaming doesn't destroy nutrients to the same extent as frying, and only a small amount of oil (if any) is needed.

Use a shallow pan or a deep frying pan with a thick base and a lid that seals well. First, add 2 tbsp of liquid to the pan, whether water, vegetable stock or a watered-down sauce. Once it boils, immediately add some vegetables, sauté rapidly for a minute or two then turn up the heat. Add 1–2 tbsp more of the liquid and put the lid on tightly. After 1 minute, add the rest of the ingredients. Then turn the heat down after 2 minutes and steam until cooked.

If you prefer, you can add 1 tsp–1 tbsp olive oil, butter or coconut oil to the pan, warm it, add the ingredients and then sauté. After a couple of minutes, add 2 tbsp of liquid as above and put the lid on. Steam until done, keeping vegetables al dente.

Waterless cooking
Special pans can be bought, in which you can 'boil' foods by steaming them in their own juice and 'fry' foods with no oil. Either method is excellent for preserving both nutrients and flavour.

Baking
Although baking is a useful technique, bear in mind that the higher the temperature and the longer you cook something, the higher the GL becomes. Avoid coating food with oil, as it is unnecessary, and the oil has a negative effect on your body.

Grilling
Grilling foods that contain fat is less damaging than frying. Browned or burnt food, however, has the potential to cause damage to your health. Try to avoid barbecued food, or at least ensure that what you eat is not charred.

Frying
Keep frying to a minimum, and avoid deep-frying altogether. When you do fry, use small amounts of coconut oil or olive oil rather than vegetable oils.

Microwaving
Using the microwave to cook foods is not the ideal choice as it destroys more nutrients than if they are steamed. If you must microwave, it is better to use the lower-voltage/heat settings for longer. Cover dishes to encourage steaming, although you do need to leave some room for steam to escape. The temperatures reached in fat particles are very high, so avoid microwaving oily

fish, as it will destroy the essential fats it contains. Do also remember that microwave ovens give off electromagnetic radiation up to six feet away.

USEFUL UTENSILS

There are few must-have utensils needed to cook the low-GL way, although reliable weighing scales are invaluable for accurate measurement of ingredients and portion sizes. A steamer is also a must, although it doesn't matter whether you use a saucepan with a steamer insert or an electric steamer. A handheld blender and a food processor are useful time-savers, but by no means essential. You'll also need a seed grinder (a redundant coffee grinder could be used here).

Special note
Recipes are for either one or two people, as marked. If there's only one of you, halve the portion sizes or make enough for two meals and pop one in the fridge.

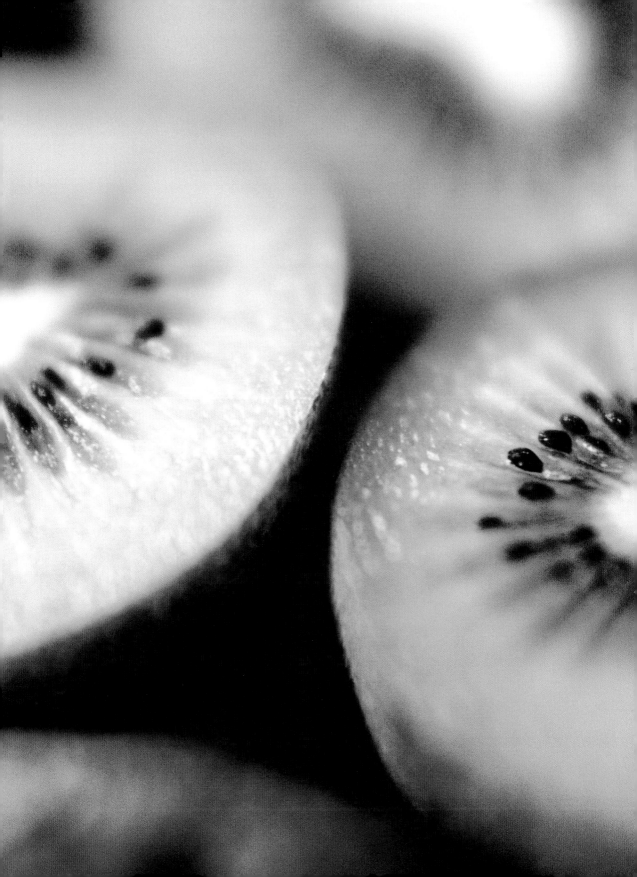

BREAKFASTS

Each of these breakfasts provides 10⑥ (or just under), to comply with the GL guidelines for main meals. They are designed to fill you up rather than fatten you. If you lack inspiration or energy in the morning, the Low-GL Get Up & Go is a great solution (see page 62). It is a blend of powdered whole foods and nutrients, which just needs to be mixed with milk and fruit for a filling breakfast smoothie.

Low-GL breakfast tips

⤍ Your lowest-GL choices are oat flakes or porridge made with milk or water, sprinkled with berries and ground mixed seeds; or toasted rye or wholemeal bread with a poached egg.
⤍ Protein foods such as dairy products have a minimal GL score, leaving you with 5⑥ for cereal and another for fruit.
⤍ Eggs, meat and fish contain virtually no carbohydrate at all, so they have a GL of 0, again leaving you with 10⑥ for bread.

Porridge

Oats are full of soluble fibre for healthy digestion and release their energy very slowly to keep you filled up all the way through to your snack and lunchtime.

SERVES 1
35g (1¹/₄oz) whole porridge oats
225ml (8fl oz) water (the guide is two parts water to one part oats)
1 tbsp seeds (such as any combination of pre-cracked linseeds, sunflower, sesame and pumpkin seeds)
A little xylitol to sweeten or a sprinkling of Solo or other low-sodium salt, to taste (optional)

1 Place the oats and water in a pan. Bring to the boil then gently simmer, stirring, until the porridge thickens and the oats soften.
2 Stir the seeds into the porridge and spoon into a bowl.
3 Sprinkle with xylitol or the salt, if using.

MAINTENANCE PHASE (PER PERSON) ✓
add a sliced banana instead of the fruit suggested above, or increase the oats serving size to 50g (1³/₄oz), or have one slice of pumpernickel-style rye bread or medium-sliced wholemeal toast with nut butter as well

COOK'S NOTES
Serving suggestion (per person)
a chopped apple or pear, or 2 plums or apricots, or a couple of handfuls of berries
Variations
sprinkle with ground cinnamon and/or ginger. Use nuts instead of seeds or omit entirely
Allergy suitability
wheat, dairy and yeast free
vegan

One-minute muesli

This combination of oats, nuts and seeds can be thrown together in an instant, or, if you get organised, make up a batch to see you through the week. The oats make this easier to digest than wheat-based muesli, plus the nuts and seeds make it rich in protein, minerals and essential fats. Sweeten it with xylitol if you like.

SERVES 1
50g (1³/₄oz) whole oat flakes
3 tbsp mixed nuts and/or seeds (such as ground or flaked almonds, pecan nuts, walnuts or hazelnuts, pumpkin, sunflower, sesame or flax seeds)
1 heaped tsp xylitol (optional)

Shake or stir the ingredients together until well mixed.

MAINTENANCE PHASE (PER PERSON) ✓
have a sliced banana instead of the fruit suggestions above, or have a slice of pumpernickel-style rye bread or medium-sliced wholemeal toast with nut butter as well

COOK'S NOTES
Serving suggestion (per person)
¹/₂ x 150g (5¹/₂oz) punnet of berries (or chopped apple or pear, or 2 plums or apricots) and a couple of tablespoons of live natural yogurt, soya yogurt, skimmed milk, soya milk or nut milk
Allergy suitability
wheat, dairy and yeast free
vegan
Storage instructions
you can make up a large batch and store in an airtight container

Scrambled eggs on toast

Comfort food that is also very quick to make. Eggs are packed with zinc for healthy skin and a strong immune system.

SERVES 1
2 medium organic or free range eggs
Freshly ground black pepper
2 slices rye bread or 1 medium slice wholemeal bread
1 tsp coconut oil or olive oil
Freshly ground black pepper

1 Beat the eggs together with the pepper.
2 Toast the bread.
3 While the bread is toasting, heat the oil in a small pan over a gentle heat and pour in the beaten eggs.
4 Slowly stir the eggs with a wooden spoon, scraping along the base of the pan as they cook to keep them moving and help stop them sticking. Remove from the heat as soon as the eggs are almost set but still a little runny and moist. Serve on the toast.

MAINTENANCE PHASE (PER PERSON) ✅
add a handful (around 5) grilled or pan-fried cherry tomatoes or 1 large tomato (cook until the skin wrinkles)

COOK'S NOTES
Allergy suitability
wheat, dairy and yeast free (use rye bread if you cannot eat wheat, and sourdough bread if you cannot eat yeast)
vegetarian

Fruit salad with yogurt and seeds

Cool and refreshing in the summer and packed with vitamins, antioxidants and essential fats to have you brimming with health.

SERVES 1
7 🍏-worth of fruit (such as ½ apple, 2 plums and ½ punnet of berries, about 50g (1¾oz) (see Fruit Serving Sizes Chart on page 73), chopped and cored as necessary
2 tbsp live natural yogurt or soya yogurt
1 tbsp seeds (such as pumpkin seeds and sunflower seeds)

Place the fruit in a bowl, top with yogurt and scatter with seeds.

MAINTENANCE PHASE (PER PERSON) ✅
add ½ small, sliced banana to the fruit mixture, or have a piece of pumpernickel-style rye toast, or medium-sliced wholemeal toast with nut butter as well

COOK'S NOTES
Allergy suitability
gluten, wheat and dairy free (if using soya yogurt)
vegetarian
vegan (if using soya yogurt)
Storage instructions
make this fresh each day to maximise the nutrients in the fruit and stop it from discolouring. Keep chilled if you are not going to eat it immediately

Breakfast smoothie

A complete meal in a glass, blended so that you can drink it just before rushing out of the door. Vary the fruit you use (although choose low-GL ones such as apples, peaches, oranges, plums and apricots, and keep within 10ⓖ per person) to keep it interesting and to get a range of different nutrients.

SERVES 1
1 tbsp seeds (such as linseeds, pumpkin, sunflower
**   or sesame seeds) (optional)**
150g (5¹/₂oz) live, organic natural yogurt, or soya yogurt
¹/₂ banana
1 punnet of berries, about 100g (3¹/₂oz) (use frozen berries
**   when fresh ones are out of season)**
A little lemon or apple juice (if necessary)

1 Grind the seeds, if using, in a mini blender or coffee grinder.
2 Blend all the ingredients with a hand-held blender until smooth.
If it is too thick you can thin it with a little water, lemon or apple juice.

MAINTENANCE PHASE (PER PERSON) ✅
have a slice of toasted pumpernickel-style rye bread or 2 rough oatcakes with nut butter afterwards

COOK'S NOTES
Allergy suitability
gluten, wheat and dairy free
(if using soya yogurt)
vegetarian
vegan (if using soya yogurt)
Storage instruction
make this fresh each day, as the seeds make the mixture very thick if left to sit for too long. Keep chilled if you are not going to drink it immediately

Low-GL Get Up & Go

A balanced blend of all the vitamins, minerals, fibre, protein and essential fats that you need each morning to make sure you are firing on all cylinders (see Further Resources for details).

SERVES 1
300ml (10fl oz/¹/₂ pint) skimmed milk (or soya, quinoa or nut milk)
¹/₂ banana, or a punnet of berries, about 100g (3¹/₂oz)
1 serving Low-GL Get Up & Go powder

Blend milk, fruit and Get Up & Go powder until smooth.

MAINTENANCE PHASE (PER PERSON) ✅
have a slice of toasted pumpernickel-style rye bread or 2 rough oatcakes with nut butter afterwards

COOK'S NOTES
Allergy suitability
gluten, wheat and dairy free
(if using dairy-free milk)
vegetarian
vegan (if using non-dairy milk)
Storage instructions
make fresh each day. Keep chilled if you are not going to drink it immediately

Breakfast sundae

A home-made version of the fruit, yogurt and granola cups that you see in smart coffee shops and delis. This recipe uses low-GL ingredients and is free from sugar.

COOK'S NOTES
Allergy suitability
wheat and dairy free (if using soya yogurt)
vegetarian
vegan (if using soya yogurt)
Storage instructions
make this fresh each day otherwise the oats will become soggy in the yogurt

SERVES 1
1 tbsp oats
1 heaped tsp xylitol
1 heaped tsp ground almonds
$^1/_2$ banana, sliced
200g (7oz) live natural yogurt or soya yogurt

1 Mix the oats with the xylitol and almonds.
2 Put the banana slices in the bottom of a short, wide glass (or bowl), cover with yogurt then sprinkle the oat mixture on top.

MAINTENANCE PHASE (PER PERSON) ✓
add 2 chopped apples to the mixture or have a slice of toasted pumpernickel-style rye bread or 2 rough oatcakes with nut butter afterwards

Toast and nut butter

If you normally grab a piece of toast before heading out of the door, make sure it is wholegrain and top it with a spread that contains protein. Nut butter is perfect, as it means you don't have to waste time or fat on normal butter, and the nuts provide minerals and essential fats as well as protein.

COOK'S NOTES
Variations
use 4 rough oatcakes per person instead of bread
Allergy suitability
wheat and dairy free (use rye bread if wheat intolerant, and sourdough bread if you cannot eat yeast)
vegan

SERVES 1
2 slices rye bread or 1 medium slice wholemeal bread
Peanut butter, or another nut butter such as cashew, hazelnut or almond, or pumpkin-seed butter (look in health-food stores if you cannot find them in supermarkets)

Toast the bread and spread with nut butter.

MAINTENANCE PHASE (PER PERSON) ✓
top with $^1/_2$ small sliced banana, or have a 5 GL piece of fruit as well (such as an apple, pear or 2 plums or apricots)

Omelette in pitta bread

It takes just a few minutes to make an omelette, and here it is stuffed inside a pitta pocket so that it can be eaten standing up or on the run, without the need for a plate or knife and fork.

SERVES 1
2 organic or free range eggs
1 tsp coconut or olive oil
1 wholemeal pitta bread
A little salt or low-sodium salt
Freshly ground black pepper

1 Beat the eggs with the pepper and salt.
2 Place the oil in a frying pan and heat to a medium heat. Tip to coat the base.
3 Toast the pitta bread while you cook the omelette.
4 Pour the egg mixture into the pan and scrape the base slowly as the omelette cooks. When it is set on the bottom but still soft on top, loosen underneath with a spatula and fold the omelette in half.
5 Slit along one length of the toasted pitta bread and open out. Carefully tip or roll the omelette off the pan onto a plate and stuff or fold it into the pitta bread.

MAINTENANCE PHASE (PER PERSON) ✅
have a 5 GL piece of fruit (such as an apple or pear) as well

COOK'S NOTES
Variations
add a sliced tomato
Allergy suitability
dairy free
vegetarian

SNACKS

Standard snack fare is often off the GL scale. Impulse eats such as sweets, chocolate, crisps, biscuits or muffins and soft drinks are designed to give you an instant energy buzz from all that sugar or caffeine, but you soon come crashing down into an energy slump. The following snacks have been chosen specifically for their protein and carbohydrate balance and their low GL (of 5𝐆𝐋). Choose two for each day, to make up your 10 GL snack allowance. The snacks are important, as they help to keep blood sugar levels even between meals and stop you from reaching for less healthy alternatives.

Low-GL snack tips

⇢ You can eat a small apple or pear or a punnet of berries for 5𝐆𝐋, whereas bananas and dried fruit have a much higher GL.
⇢ Remember: rye bread has a much lower GL than standard wheat bread, so you can eat a whole slice of pumpernickel or sourdough rye bread for 5𝐆𝐋 but only half a slice of normal bread.
⇢ Oatcakes are another low-GL snack – you can have 3 for 5𝐆𝐋.
⇢ Protein foods such as peanut butter and hummus, or nuts, contain negligible 𝐆𝐋.

5-GL SNACKS

⇢ 2 rough oatcakes spread with hummus

⇢ 2 rough oatcakes spread with cottage cheese

⇢ 2 rough oatcakes spread with reduced fat cream cheese

⇢ 2 rough oatcakes spread with nut butter

⇢ 2 rough oatcakes spread with tuna and guacamole or salsa (optional: top with cucumber slices or cress/alfalfa sprouts)

⇢ 2 rough oatcakes spread with tuna mayo (optional: top with cucumber slices or cress/alfalfa sprouts)

⇢ 1 slice pumpernickel-style rye bread with nut butter (optional: top with cucumber slices or cress/alfalfa sprouts)

⇢ 1 slice pumpernickel-style rye bread with hummus (optional: top with cucumber slices or cress/alfalfa sprouts)

⇢ 1 slice pumpernickel-style rye bread with cottage cheese and cucumber slices

⇢ Crudités (such as pepper, cucumber, celery, cabbage or carrot sticks, sugarsnap peas, mangetouts, baby corn, radishes, spring onions) with 150g (5½oz) hummus (about ⅔ small pot)

⇢ Crudités (such as pepper, cucumber, celery, cabbage or carrot sticks, sugarsnap peas, mangetouts, baby corn, radishes, spring onions) with 120g (4¼oz) cottage cheese (about ⅔ small pot)

⇢ Crudités (such as pepper, cucumber, celery, cabbage or carrot sticks, sugarsnap peas, mangetouts, baby corn, radishes, spring onions) with 150g (5½oz) guacamole (about ⅔ small pot)

⇢ Fruit and yogurt smoothie, such as 150g (5½oz) organic live natural yogurt blended with berries, or a shop-bought one with natural yogurt and no added sugar

⇢ Live natural yogurt or cottage cheese with 5 ⒼⓁ of berries or chopped fruit

⇢ Piece of fruit (equivalent to 5 ⒼⓁ) with 2 teaspoons nuts or seeds

⇢ Miso soup (one serving, from a packet; simply mix powder with boiling water) plus a piece of fruit afterwards (equivalent to 5 ⒼⓁ)

⇢ Boiled egg with 2 rough oatcakes

⇢ Omelette (cooked as for Omelette in Pitta Bread on page 95. Roll out of pan and onto the bread) with a piece of toasted pumpernickel-style rye bread

⇢ Handful of olives plus a piece of fruit (equivalent to 5 ⒼⓁ)

See page 73 for a list of fruit serving sizes.

FOOD ON THE MOVE/WORKING LUNCHES

When you are busy or away from home it can be hard to stick to a diet or choose healthy options. So we have come up with some simple salads and sandwiches, which take a matter of minutes to throw together in the morning or the night before, for you to take with you. We have also included 'pick and mix'-style charts for salads (see pages 105-107) and sandwiches (see pages 113-115), which give options of different ingredients, and correct quantities for both the weight loss and maintenance phases. You will then easily be able to come up with your own ideas when preparing packed lunches or choosing options at the deli or sandwich bar, safe in the knowledge that you are sticking to the Holford Low-GL Diet guidelines.

Low-GL eating out tips

··➤ Skip the starter and don't feel you have to have a pudding when eating out.
··➤ Ask for dressings and sauces to be served separately.
··➤ Decide in advance to say 'no' to bread, chocolates or liqueurs.
··➤ Phone ahead and ask for a low-carb option to be added to the menu.
··➤ See the guidelines in Chapter 8 for further information.

SALADS

A salad doesn't have to mean limp lettuce, soggy tomato and curling cucumber. Add enough interesting, nutritious ingredients, such as those used in these recipes, and it turns into a tasty, satisfying main meal. Plus, it is an excellent way to incorporate plenty of raw vegetables easily into your diet, for fibre and vitamins to keep you feeling and looking in the pink.

A note on dressings
You can use 1 tbsp ready-made dressing (choose one with negligible or no added sugar) or drizzle balsamic vinegar or lemon juice and a little extra virgin olive oil on your salad to add flavour. You can also add taste without fat by adding full-flavoured ingredients like mustard, tamari or soy sauce, crushed garlic, grated ginger and fresh herbs. Bear in mind that pickles and chutneys can be heavily sweetened so go easy on them.

Chicken, sun-blush tomato and pine nut salad

A classic combination of Italian flavours that is easy to prepare.

SERVES 1
1/2 x 150g (51/2oz) bag fully prepared mixed salad leaves, organic where possible
75g (23/4oz) skinned, cooked chicken meat, or a small cooked chicken breast fillet, sliced into bite-sized pieces
2 tsp pine nuts
4 pieces sun-blush tomato, roughly chopped, or a handful of cherry tomatoes, halved
2.5cm (1in) chunk cucumber, diced
2 tbsp ready-made dressing (low in sugar or sugar-free) or a mixture of balsamic vinegar and extra virgin olive oil
Freshly ground black pepper

Mix together the salad ingredients, dressing and pepper.

MAINTENANCE PHASE (PER PERSON) ✔
increase to 90g (31/4oz) (dry weight) quinoa or serve the salad with a wholemeal pitta bread

Greek salad

One of the best salad combinations ever. It's ideal for a picnic.

SERVES 1
1 small red onion, diced
6 cherry tomatoes, halved
7.5cm (3in) chunk cucumber, diced
1 tbsp pitted black olives, roughly chopped
75g (23/4oz) feta cheese
Freshly ground black pepper

FOR THE DRESSING
1 tbsp ready-made (sugar free) vinaigrette, or mix together:
    1 tbsp extra virgin olive oil, 2 tsp white wine vinegar,
    1/2 tsp dried oregano, freshly ground black pepper

1 Combine the vegetables and olives, add the dressing and toss.
2 Crumble the feta over the top and lightly toss through the vegetables.
3 Season with black pepper and chill lightly or serve immediately.

MAINTENANCE PHASE (PER PERSON) ✔
replace pulses or potatoes with 1 wholemeal pitta bread

Tuna and tomato salad

Try this lower fat, more interesting alternative to tuna mayo. The butterbeans not only add flavour and texture to the dish but they also provide fibre and hormone-balancing phytoestrogens.

SERVES 1
1/2 x 410g (14¹/2oz) can butterbeans, drained and rinsed
1/2 x 400g (14oz) can chopped tomatoes in tomato juice (get the best quality you can find)
1/2 red onion, finely sliced or diced
1/2 x 185g (6¹/2oz) can tuna, drained (140g (5oz) drained weight)
Sprinkle of herbed salt (if you can find it), or use sea salt or low-sodium salt plus 1/2 tsp dried mixed herbs or Italian mixed herbs (herbs are optional)
1/2 x 150g (5¹/2oz) bag fully prepared salad leaves, organic where possible, or 75g (2³/4oz) lettuce
Freshly ground black pepper

1 Place the beans, tomatoes, onion and tuna in a bowl. Mix together and season to taste with herbed salt and pepper.
2 Spoon on top of the salad.

MAINTENANCE PHASE (PER PERSON) ✅
add 3 sun-blush tomato pieces to the tuna mixture

COOK'S NOTES
Variations
add 1 tbsp chopped pitted olives to the mixture, if you like. Vegetarians could replace the tuna with 100g (3¹/2oz) cubed smoked tofu
Allergy suitability
gluten, wheat and dairy free

Goat's cheese, pear and pecan salad

A brilliant combination of flavours that is very simple to fling together.

SERVES 1
1 slice firm goat's cheese (approximately 75–100g/2³/4–3¹/2oz), sliced or crumbled into chunks
1 ripe pear, cored and thinly sliced
1 tbsp pecan halves (roughly chopped, if you prefer)
1 Little Gem lettuce, washed and drained, and torn into bite-sized pieces
A couple of good handfuls of watercress, roughly chopped or torn

Scatter the cheese, pear slices and nuts over a bed of lettuce and watercress. The fat and flavour from the nuts and cheese mean that you shouldn't need extra dressing.

MAINTENANCE PHASE (PER PERSON) ✅
increase to 4 rough oatcakes

COOK'S NOTES
Serving suggestion (per person)
with 2 rough oatcakes or 1 slice pumpernickel-style rye bread
Variations
use a small apple instead of the pear. Replace the pecan nuts with walnut halves. Add a celery stick, sliced, if you like
Allergy suitability
gluten and wheat free
vegetarian

Salade niçoise

You can make this celebrated French classic salad as quick or
as complicated as you like. If you have time, do include the capers
and spring onions, as they add so much to the overall flavour.

SERVES 1
$1/2$ x 185g ($6^1/_2$oz) can or jar of tuna, drained (140g (5oz) drained)
$1/2$ Romaine lettuce or 2 Little Gem lettuces, washed well,
      dried and torn into bite-sized pieces
3 spring onions, sliced on the diagonal (optional)
3 pitted black olives, roughly chopped
1 tsp capers, well rinsed (optional)
1 egg, hard-boiled for 8 minutes, shelled and chopped into
      smallish chunks
2 anchovies in oil, drained on kitchen paper (optional)
6 cherry tomatoes, halved
$1/2$ x 410g ($14^1/_2$oz) can mixed pulses, drained and rinsed
$1/2$ x 225g (8oz) can cooked French green beans, drained and
      rinsed well to remove any salty water
Freshly ground black pepper

FOR THE DRESSING
1 tbsp ready-made vinaigrette

1 Toss all the salad ingredients together.
2 Pour over the dressing and toss again, gently.

MAINTENANCE PHASE (PER PERSON) ✓
serve with 3 small boiled baby new potatoes (in addition to the
mixed pulses)

Smoked salmon with cottage cheese salad

The creamy, mild flavour of cottage cheese goes beautifully with the salty, sweet salmon. This dish is rich in essential fats from the oily salmon, and low in saturated fat, as cottage cheese is virtually fat-free.

SERVES 1

1/2 x 150g (5¹/₂oz) bag fully prepared mixed salad leaves,
    organic where possible
2.5cm (1in) chunk cucumber, finely sliced
125g (4¹/₂oz) cottage cheese
1/2 x 75g (2³/₄oz) pack smoked salmon, torn into strips
1 tbsp lemon juice
Freshly ground black pepper

1 Place the leaves and cucumber on a plate. Put the cottage cheese and salmon on top.
2 Drizzle with lemon juice and season with plenty of black pepper.

MAINTENANCE PHASE (PER PERSON) ✅

serve with 2 slices of pumpernickel-style rye bread or 5 rough oatcakes

COOK'S NOTES
Serving suggestion (per person)
3 rough oatcakes or 1 slice pumpernickel-style rye bread
Variations
use the same weight of smoked trout, mackerel or cooked prawns instead of salmon. Vegetarians could replace the salmon with 1 tbsp pumpkin seeds per person
Allergy suitability
wheat free

Mackerel and chickpea salad

Strongly flavoured mackerel is an oily fish that is a rich source of omega-3 essential fats, which are required for skin, hormones and brain function. Its rich flavour works well with the salty olive tapenade and the mild chickpeas.

SERVES 1

1/2 x 225g (8oz) jar or can mackerel fillets in oil, drained and placed
    on kitchen paper to absorb excess oil (160g (5³/₄oz) drained weight)
1/2 x 410g (14¹/₂oz) can chickpeas
1 tbsp tapenade
1/2 x 150g (5¹/₂oz) bag fully prepared baby or young leaf spinach,
    organic where possible, finely sliced or shredded
1 celery stick, finely sliced (optional)
2.5cm (1in) chunk cucumber, diced (optional)

Tip all the ingredients in a bowl and mix so that the fish flakes and everything else becomes coated in tapenade.

MAINTENANCE PHASE (PER PERSON) ✅

add 50g (1³/₄oz) (dry weight) quinoa or a toasted mini wholemeal pitta bread

COOK'S NOTES
Variations
use pitted black olives instead of tapenade (in which case you could use 1 tbsp per person of the olives' marinating oil to dress the salad). Use butterbeans or cannellini beans instead of the chickpeas. Use chopped watercress instead of the spinach
Allergy suitability
gluten, wheat and dairy free

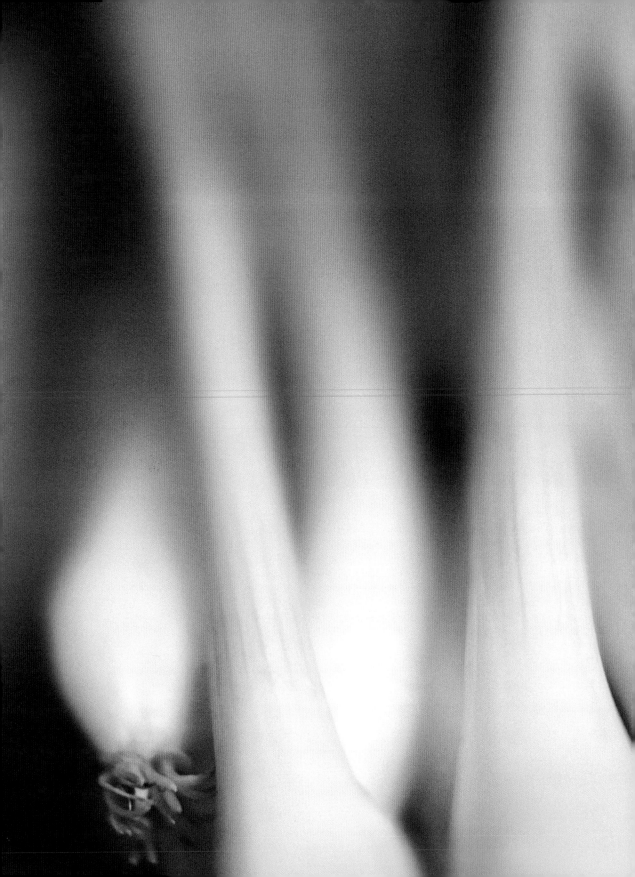

MIX-AND-MATCH SALADS

If you fancy creating your own 'superfood' salad, you can use the table on pages 106–7 to pick and mix your own ingredients, either at home or when you are choosing lunch from a deli or salad bar. To get a 10Ⓖ meal you can fill your plate with vegetables from the 'Unlimited' box then select one of the options from both the 'Choose 1 Protein' and 'Choose 1 Carbohydrate' boxes, to provide a balanced meal of protein, carbohydrate and plenty of fibrous vegetables.

For example, you could have spinach, watercress, rocket, cherry tomatoes, artichoke hearts and olives, with chicken slices and butterbeans. Alternatively, try Romaine lettuce, spring onions, celery, roasted red peppers, and smoked mackerel flaked through with quinoa. The serving sizes here are for one person, and include maintenance phase portions when you are allowed more carbohydrate to bring your meal up to 15Ⓖ.

UNLIMITED

Salad leaves

Lettuce or other leaves, such as spinach, watercress, rocket

Other non-starchy vegetables

Vegetables, such as spring onions or red onion, cherry tomatoes, cucumber, radishes, diced peppers, beansprouts, celery, fresh herbs, vegetable antipasti (such as marinated artichoke hearts, roasted peppers or olives – drain off any excess oil)

CHOOSE 1

Protein

1 chicken breast fillet or equivalent slices or strips of chicken, turkey or lean ham

85g (3oz) (medium fillet) smoked fish, such as smoked salmon, trout or mackerel

85g (3oz) (6 large) cooked prawns

½ x 85g (3oz) can tuna

120g (4¼oz) cottage cheese

75g (2¾oz) cheese, such as feta or goat's cheese

2 hard-boiled eggs (or mash 1 hard-boiled egg into 1 tbsp cottage cheese)

1 tbsp nuts or seeds, such as pine nuts, pecan nuts, walnuts, cashew nuts or pumpkin seeds

200g (7oz) hummus (small pot)

65g (2¼oz) quinoa (dry weight)

100g (3½oz) smoked tofu, cubed

CHOOSE 1

Carbohydrate
(grains and starchy vegetables)

1 medium carrot (grated) or apple (diced)
maintenance phase: 1 large carrot or apple

110g (3¾oz) beetroot
maintenance phase: 160g (5¾oz)

½ x 410g (14½oz) can (2 tbsp) mixed pulses, butterbeans, lentils or chickpeas (or other pulse)
maintenance phase: ²/₃ x 410g (14½oz) can (3 heaped tbsp)

3 rough oatcakes
maintenance phase: 5 rough oatcakes

¾ wholemeal pitta bread (or to make life easier, have a whole pitta bread for 10 but don't have it with a carbohydrate containing filling – so no sun-dried tomatoes or hummus, for example
maintenance phase: 1 pitta

1½ slices rye bread
maintenance phase: 2 slices rye bread

65g (2¼oz) quinoa (dry weight)
maintenance phase: 90g (3¼oz) (very large serving)

40g (1½oz) brown basmati rice (dry weight) (very small serving)
maintenance phase: 60g (2¼oz) (small serving)

40g (1½oz) wholemeal pasta (dry weight) (medium serving)
maintenance phase: 55g (2oz) (medium-large serving)

3 small baby new potatoes
maintenance phase: 4 small baby new potatoes

½ small baked potato/sweet potato
maintenance phase: 1 small baked potato/sweet potato

SANDWICHES

If you are grabbing lunch on the run or having to buy something when out, sandwiches are quick and convenient, but remember that many shop-bought sandwiches will use high GL, thick-sliced white bread or enormous rolls or bagels, taking you well over your 10GL goal per meal. If you can, stick to thin-sliced wholemeal bread or rye bread, and go for open sandwiches using one slice of bread (or the bottom half of a roll or bagel), to cut down on the GL load. A protein-rich filling or topping should ensure you feel full up, and you can always eat plenty of salad.

Smoked trout sandwich with tapenade and watercress

This sandwich is always popular. Sliced into small squares it makes for simple but sophisticated canapés or drinks party nibbles, or serve it whole for a filling lunch that is packed with essential fats (from the fish) and vitamin C (from the watercress).

SERVES 1
2 tsp tapenade, or to taste
1¹/₂ slices pumpernickel-style rye bread
1 smoked trout fillet, about 75g (2³/₄oz), skinned, flaked and checked for bones
1 handful watercress, well chopped

1 Spread the tapenade thinly over the bread then spread the flaked fish on top.
2 Scatter watercress over and season with black pepper. Cut the sandwich in half.

MAINTENANCE PHASE (PER PERSON) ✔
increase to 2 slices pumpernickel-style rye bread (or 5 oatcakes)

COOK'S NOTES
Variations
replace the pumpernickel-style rye bread with 3 rough oatcakes per person
Storage instructions
eat the same day
Allergy suitability
wheat free

Hummus and roasted pepper wrap

Buy ready-made hummus from the supermarket or deli for an instant sandwich filling. You could also use roasted red pepper hummus, available from most supermarkets, instead of adding roasted red peppers separately (as these can be quite expensive when bought in a jar from the deli).

SERVES 1
1 small tortilla wrap
1 heaped tbsp hummus
1 tbsp roasted pepper pieces (from a jar or the deli)
1 handful lettuce, spinach, rocket or watercress
2.5cm (1in) chunk cucumber, finely sliced
Freshly ground black pepper

Spread the hummus down the centre of the wrap, place the peppers and salad on top, season and roll up.

MAINTENANCE PHASE (PER PERSON) ✔
increase to 1 large wrap, 2 slices pumpernickel-style rye bread or 5 oatcakes

COOK'S NOTES
Variations
replace the wrap with 1¹/₂ slices pumpernickel-style rye bread or 3 rough oatcakes per person. Replace the hummus with guacamole, or 75g (2³/₄oz) cooked and sliced skinless chicken or turkey
Storage instructions
eat the same day
Allergy suitability
dairy free
vegan

Ham, artichoke heart and tomato open sandwich

Although a red meat, ham is not necessarily a high-fat choice if you choose a lean, unprocessed kind. Here it is served with the unusual addition of marinated artichoke hearts, which add flavour and moisture without the need for butter, but you could also use cream cheese if you cannot get hold of artichoke hearts (it is also much cheaper).

SERVES 1
2 marinated artichoke heart pieces, drained (in jars or fresh from
    the deli) (or 1 heaped tbsp reduced-fat cream cheese)
1¹/₂ slices pumpernickel-style rye bread
1 ripe tomato, sliced
4 large, thin slices (or enough to cover the bread) lean, unprocessed ham
Freshly ground black pepper
Couple of basil leaves, roughly torn, to garnish (optional)

1 Squash the artichoke hearts onto the bread. Lay the tomato slices and ham on top.
2 Season with black pepper and scatter with basil, if using.

MAINTENANCE PHASE (PER PERSON) ✔
increase to 2 slices rye bread (or 5 oatcakes)

COOK'S NOTES
Variations
replace the rye bread with 3 rough oatcakes per person. Replace the ham with turkey, chicken, pastrami or smoked fish. Omit the artichokes and use pesto or mustard and gherkins to add moisture and flavour
Storage instructions
eat the same day
Allergy suitability
wheat free

Smoked salmon and cream cheese on rye bread

The classic pairing of smoked salmon and cream cheese is not only delicious but is also very quick to make. This sandwich is high in heart-helping essential fats and low in artery-clogging saturated fat.

SERVES 1
1 tbsp low-fat cream cheese
1¹/₂ slices pumpernickel-style rye bread
2.5cm (1in) chunk cucumber, finely sliced
75g (2³/₄oz) smoked salmon, about 3 slices
Freshly ground black pepper

Spread the cream cheese over the bread, cover with cucumber slices then lay the salmon slices on top. Season with black pepper.

MAINTENANCE PHASE (PER PERSON) ✔
increase to 2 slices pumpernickel-style rye bread (or 5 oatcakes)

COOK'S NOTES
Variations
replace the pumpernickel-style rye bread with 3 rough oatcakes per person. Use cottage cheese instead of cream cheese, or 1 tbsp tapenade or pesto. Use roughly chopped watercress instead of cucumber
Storage instructions
eat the same day
Allergy suitability
wheat free

Low-fat egg 'mayo' on oatcakes

Our version of egg 'mayo' uses low-fat cottage cheese instead of mayonnaise to bind the mixture. The added protein from the cottage cheese makes it more filling and less oily.

SERVES 1
1 large egg, hard-boiled for 8 minutes and peeled
2 tbsp cottage cheese
Pinch of salt or low-sodium salt (optional, if needed)
3 rough oatcakes
6 thin cucumber slices or 1 tbsp cress or alfalfa sprouts
Freshly ground black pepper

1 Mash the egg with the cottage cheese and season to taste.
2 When ready for lunch, spread the oatcakes with the egg mixture and top with cucumber, cress or alfalfa sprouts.

MAINTENANCE PHASE (PER PERSON) ✔
increase to 5 rough oatcakes (or 2 slices rye bread)

COOK'S NOTES
Serving suggestion (per person)
with some salad if wished
Variations
replace the oatcakes with
1¹/₂ slices pumpernickel-style
rye bread per person
Storage instructions
keep the egg mixture chilled until
ready to use (it keeps well for up
to 2 days)
Allergy suitability
wheat free
vegetarian

Deli-style pastrami open rye sandwich

If you love high-GL bagels and burgers this American-style sandwich should appeal. Pastrami is incredibly lean but full of flavour.

SERVES 1
A little coarse-grain mustard (optional)
1¹/₂ thin slices pumpernickel-style rye bread
A couple of gherkins, thinly sliced (optional)
75g (2³/₄oz) pastrami, bresaola or lean, unprocessed ham slices
1 small, ripe tomato, thinly sliced
Freshly ground black pepper

1 Spread the mustard, if using, thinly over the bread, and add the gherkins (if using).
2 Cover with the meat slices and top with tomato. Season with black pepper.

MAINTENANCE PHASE (PER PERSON) ✔
increase to 2 slices rye bread (or 5 oatcakes)

COOK'S NOTES
Serving suggestion (per person)
a mixed salad
Variations
replace the pumpernickel-style
rye bread with 3 rough oatcakes
per person. Use chicken or turkey
slices instead of pastrami,
bresaola or ham. Use roughly
chopped watercress or rocket
instead of tomato
Storage instructions
eat the same day
Allergy suitability
wheat free

Greek stuffed pitta bread

A Greek salad-inspired filling, with plenty of flavour from the feta cheese and olives.

SERVES 1
75g (2³/₄oz) feta cheese, cubed
3 pitted black olives, halved
3 cherry tomatoes, halved
1/4 red onion, diced
2.5cm (1in) chunk cucumber, diced
1 handful lettuce
1/4 tsp dried oregano (optional)
1 wholemeal pitta bread, toasted and one edge cut open

Mix together all of the salad ingredients and stuff into the pitta bread.

MAINTENANCE PHASE (PER PERSON) ✓
have a side salad as well

MIX-AND-MATCH SANDWICHES

On the pages that follow are some more options to help you to create delicious, low-GL sandwiches to keep you within your 10℗ goal per meal. Choose the type of bread you want from the 'Choose 1 Bread' box, then decide which topping and salad to put with it from the 'Choose 1 Filling' and 'Unlimited' boxes. You can also choose anything from the 'Optional' box.

So, for example, you could go for wholemeal bread and smoked salmon with rocket and pesto or an open rye-bread sandwich of cottage or cream cheese with spinach and sliced or mashed avocado. Alternatively, try a wholemeal pitta stuffed with pastrami, bresaola or lean, unprocessed ham with sliced gherkins and tomatoes, lettuce and coarse-grain mustard.

You'll notice that we haven't included butter – try to cut down on saturated fat by choosing a moist filling so that you don't notice the absence of a fatty spread. If you do want to use it, have just a thin smear, or use a little hummus or mustard instead. The serving sizes here are for one person.

CHOOSE 1

Bread (carbohydrate)

1 medium slice wholemeal bread
maintenance phase: 1 thick slice

3/4 wholemeal pitta bread (or to make life easier, have a whole pitta bread for 10 GL but don't have it with a carbohydrate-containing filling – so no sun-dried tomatoes or hummus, for example)
maintenance phase: 1 pitta

1½ slices pumpernickel-style rye bread
maintenance phase: 2 slices

3 rough oatcakes
maintenance phase: 5

1 small wrap
maintenance phase: 1½ small wraps (or 1 large)

CHOOSE 1

Filling/topping (protein)

200g (7oz) hummus (small tub)

120g (4¼oz) cottage cheese, (about ½ tub)

85g (3oz) smoked fish (a medium fillet), such as salmon, trout or mackerel

50g (1¾oz) cooked meat (couple of slices), such as chicken, turkey, ham off the bone, pastrami or bresaola

70g (2½oz) tuna ½ x 185g (6½oz) can), drained

1 tbsp taramasalata

85g (3oz) (6 large) cooked prawns

2 hard-boiled eggs (or mix 1 egg with 1 tbsp cottage cheese for a low-fat alternative to egg mayo)

1 tbsp nut butter (try hazelnut, almond or pumpkin-seed as well as peanut butter

100g (3½oz) thinly sliced smoked tofu

UNLIMITED

Salad (either in the salad or on the side)

Lettuce, rocket, spinach, watercress, tomatoes (cherry tomatoes have the lowest GL), cucumber, gherkins, spring onion or thinly sliced red onion, finely shredded cabbage.

Vegetable antipasti, such as roasted peppers or marinated artichoke hearts, drained of oil, or roasted vegetables.

Cress or other sprouted seeds (alfalfa sprouts taste similar to cress and are packed with phyto – or plant – nutrients)

OPTIONAL

Condiments for added flavour

Slick of mustard

Up to 1 tbsp tomato salsa

Up to 2 tsp pesto

Up to 2 tsp nut butter

Up to 2 tsp guacamole or sliced or mashed avocado

Up to 2 tsp tapenade

Scraping of butter

Up to 2 tsp reduced-fat cream cheese

MAIN MEALS

Each of these dishes provides 10GL (taking into account serving suggestions). They include meat, fish and vegetarian options, and are all easy and quick to prepare and cook.

Low-GL main meal tips

···❯ Remember to combine carbohydrate with protein at every meal and snack.
···❯ Buy foods as fresh and unprocessed as possible and eat them soon afterwards.
···❯ Quinoa is a good source of protein as well as carbohydrate, so it can be used as protein and/or carbohydrate in a dish.

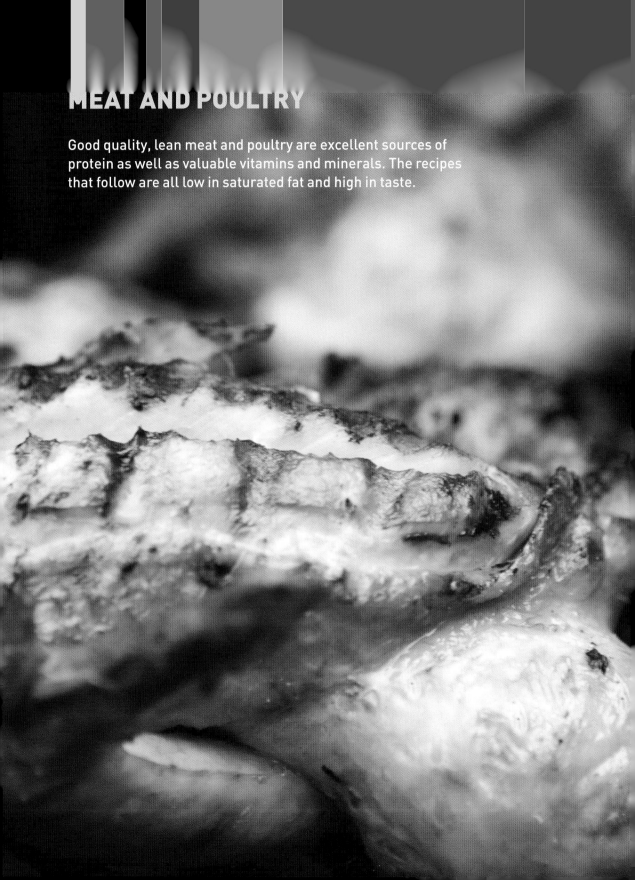

MEAT AND POULTRY

Good quality, lean meat and poultry are excellent sources of protein as well as valuable vitamins and minerals. The recipes that follow are all low in saturated fat and high in taste.

Sausage and pepper casserole

Look for good-quality, lean sausages with a high meat content, and avoid ones that are full of additives and fillers.

SERVES 2
3 peppers (mixed colours), seeded and sliced
1 red onion, sliced into long strips
2 tbsp tomato purée
1x 400g can chopped tomatoes
4 sausages
A little sea salt or low-sodium salt
Freshly ground black pepper

1 Preheat the oven to 190°C/375°F/Gas 5.
2 Place the sliced peppers and onion into a shallow casserole, stir in the tomato purée and the chopped tomatoes and season with a little salt. Put the sausages on top.
3 Bake for around an hour or until the sausages are cooked, turning halfway through to colour on both sides.
4 Season generously with black pepper.

MAINTENANCE PHASE (PER PERSON) ✔
have a small baked potato or 3–4 medium new potatoes

COOK'S NOTES
Serving suggestion (per person)
1/2 small baked potato or sweet potato, or 3 small boiled baby new potatoes, and a green salad, if you like
Variations
omit the onion and replace with another pepper. Add a teaspoon of mixed dried herbs
Storage instructions
you can prepare this in advance and keep chilled for a day until ready to cook, or keep leftovers chilled for up to 3 days
Allergy suitability
dairy free (if you cannot eat gluten or wheat, choose gluten-free sausages)

Pork chops with a mustard and crème fraîche sauce

Very quick and easy to cook; the creamy sauce can be made in seconds.

SERVES 2
2 pork chops, about 175g (6oz) each
Oil, for brushing
1 tbsp coarse-grain mustard
2 tbsp low-fat crème fraîche
A little sea salt or low-sodium salt
Freshly ground black pepper

1 Preheat the grill to high and brush the chops with a little oil then season with plenty of black pepper and a little salt.
2 Grill for around 5–10 minutes each side, or until the meat is cooked.
3 Place the mustard and crème fraîche in a small pan and stir together, heating for a couple of minutes to let the sauce combine.

MAINTENANCE PHASE (PER PERSON) ✔
have a whole small baked potato or 4 small baby new potatoes

COOK'S NOTES
Serving suggestion (per person)
3 tbsp peas and 3 small boiled baby new potatoes or 1/2 x 410g (141/2oz) can flageolet beans, rinsed and gently heated. Cut the fat from the chops before serving
Variations
use wilted spring greens or Savoy cabbage instead of peas. Swap the chops for 2 sausages per person
Allergy suitability
gluten and wheat free

Sausages with sweet potato mash and onion gravy

Bangers-and-mash comfort food is still allowed on the Holford Low-GL Diet. We have used sweet potatoes, as they mash down to a naturally creamy consistency without the need to add extra butter or milk, reducing the fat content.

SERVES 2
4 good-quality sausages with a high meat content, pricked with a fork to release the fat
1 medium–large sweet potato, peeled
1/2 tsp Marigold Reduced Salt Vegetable Bouillon powder or sea salt
Freshly ground black pepper

FOR THE GRAVY
1 tsp coconut oil or olive oil
2 onions (red or white), finely sliced
1 tsp cornflour
200ml (7fl oz/1/3 pint) vegetable stock (such as 2 tsp Marigold Reduced Salt Vegetable Bouillon powder added to 200ml (7fl oz/1/3 pint) boiling water)
1 tsp tamari or soy sauce

1 Grill or oven-cook the sausages according to the packet instructions.
2 Meanwhile, slice the sweet potato thinly and steam for 12 minutes, or until soft.
3 Place the sweet potato in a pan and mash, then stir in the bouillon powder and seasoning, and keep warm while you make the gravy.
4 Heat the oil in a saucepan and sauté the onions for 5 minutes, or until soft. Place the cornflour in a small bowl or cup and stir in the vegetable stock. Pour over the onions and simmer, stirring, for a few minutes, or until thickened.
5 Stir in the tamari or soy sauce. Check the flavour and consistency (you can add a little more tamari or water if wished, or simmer to reduce the gravy to intensify the flavour).
6 Place the sausages and mash on plates and pour the gravy over the top.

MAINTENANCE PHASE (PER PERSON) ✔
increase to 1 small–medium sweet potato

COOK'S NOTES
Variations
replace the onion with a large leek. Add a crushed garlic clove to the gravy and sauté with the onions, or add 1 teaspoon mixed dried herbs
Storage instructions
you can prepare all the components of this dish in advance and keep chilled for up to 3 days
Allergy suitability
dairy free (if you cannot eat gluten or wheat, choose gluten-free sausages)

Chicken with aubergine and peppers

A rich, warming stew of Mediterranean flavours. This dish featured in *The Holford Low-GL Diet Cookbook* and was so well received that we had to include it here. Fortunately, it is very simple to make.

SERVES 2
1 tbsp coconut oil or olive oil
2 chicken breast fillets, trimmed of fat and skin, and sliced into strips
2 garlic cloves, crushed
2 tsp ground cumin
2 large red onions, diced
1 red pepper, diced
½ medium aubergine, diced
1 tsp Marigold Reduced Salt Vegetable Bouillon powder
200g (7oz) tomato passata
Freshly ground black pepper
1 tbsp fresh basil leaves, roughly torn, to garnish (optional)

1 Heat the oil in a frying pan and sear the chicken strips on all sides, then remove from the pan and set to one side.
2 Add the garlic and cumin to the pan and fry for 30 seconds or so before adding the onions and pepper. Cook this mixture for 1 minute.
3 Tip in the aubergine and sauté gently for 5 minutes, or until all the vegetables soften.
4 Return the chicken to the pan with the bouillon powder and passata, and simmer for 10–15 minutes, or until the meat is cooked through.
5 Season with black pepper and sprinkle with basil, if using, before serving.

MAINTENANCE PHASE (PER PERSON) ✔
increase the pasta serving to 55g (2oz) or serve with a whole baked potato

Chicken and vegetable steam-fry with brown basmati rice

Steam-frying, like stir-frying, is a convenient cooking method when time is short. It is also an excellent way to enjoy a good selection of vegetables as well as eating a range of different colours, which will optimise your intake of nutrients. Steam-frying is a gentler way of cooking than the harsh, high temperature of a stir-fry, as it par-steams the food in a little liquid added to a covered wok. This way you cook the food gently to retain more nutrients without any loss of flavour.

SERVES 2
2 tsp coconut oil or olive oil

1 packet of chicken goujons, or 2 chicken breast fillets, skinned and trimmed of fat, cut into strips

1 bag pre-prepared stir-fry vegetables, or equivalent fresh vegetables, such as beansprouts, julienned (finely sliced lengthways into matchsticks), carrot, peppers, spring onions and cabbage or Chinese leaves

1 tbsp tamari or soy sauce

1 tbsp water, lemon juice, vegetable bouillon liquid or Mirin

1 Heat the oil in a wok or large saucepan and tip to coat the base.

2 Add the chicken and brown on all sides for a few minutes.

3 Add the vegetables to the pan with the liquid and immediately cover the wok with a lid to allow the ingredients to cook in the steam inside. (If you don't have a lid you can improvise by soaking a couple of sheets of kitchen paper in cold water and placing them over the food in the wok to cover it, allowing the water to create moisture in the pan.)

4 Check after a couple of minutes, stir and add a splash more water if necessary. Continue cooking until the meat and vegetables are ready (the vegetables should still be fairly crunchy to the bite).

MAINTENANCE PHASE (PER PERSON) ✅
increase to 65g (2¹/₄oz) (dry weight) brown basmati rice

COOK'S NOTES
Serving suggestion (per person)
40g (1¹/₂oz) (dry weight) brown basmati rice

Variations
serve with 65g (2¹/₄oz) (dry weight) quinoa instead of rice. Vary the vegetables used. Replace the chicken with turkey or 100g (3¹/₂oz) tofu

Storage instructions
best eaten fresh

Allergy suitability
gluten (if using tanari – wheat-free soy sauce), wheat and dairy free

Chicken with cherry tomatoes and crème fraîche

A firm favourite from *The Holford Low-GL Diet Cookbook*, this dish is not only delicious but also ridiculously simple. The tomatoes cook down to release their juice which, when combined with the crème fraîche, makes a deliciously creamy sauce.

SERVES 2
2 tbsp olive oil
2 chicken breast fillets, trimmed of fat and skin
225g (8oz) cherry tomatoes
1¹/₂ tbsp low-fat crème fraîche
1 tbsp basil leaves, chopped or roughly torn (optional)

1 Preheat the oven to 200°C/400°F/Gas 6.
2 Pour the oil into a shallow flameproof and ovenproof dish, and add the chicken breasts, turning to coat in the oil.
3 Place the whole cherry tomatoes around the chicken in the dish and cook in the oven for 50–60 minutes, or until the chicken is cooked through, basting occasionally.
4 Place the dish on the hob and add the crème fraîche. Heat gently until it starts to bubble, then simmer for a moment until the sauce thickens.
5 Stir in the basil, if using.

MAINTENANCE PHASE (PER PERSON) ✔
increase to 4 small boiled baby new potatoes or 1 small baked potato and a large green salad

COOK'S NOTES
Serving suggestion (per person)
3 small boiled baby new potatoes or half a small–medium baked potato and a green salad
Variations
use salmon fillets instead of chicken (cook at 190°C/375°F/Gas 5 for 25 minutes)
Storage instructions
better eaten fresh, but you could chill leftovers and reheat thoroughly the next day
Allergy suitability
gluten and wheat free

Fajitas

This recipe includes a version for using chicken and a vegan version that uses red kidney or black-eyed beans. Whichever way you choose to serve them, fajitas are easy to make and very tasty.

SERVES 2
2 red onions, sliced
1 garlic clove, crushed (optional)
1 red and 1 yellow pepper, seeded and sliced lengthways into strips
1 tsp coconut oil or olive oil
$2/3$ tbsp fajita seasoning (dried spices available in packets from supermarkets)
2 chicken breast fillets, skinned and cut into slices or 1 x 410g (14$1/2$oz) can red kidney or black-eyed beans, drained and rinsed
4 tsp tomato salsa (from the chiller cabinet or deli) and/or 4 tsp guacamole (from the chiller cabinet or deli)
2 small flour tortillas (wheat or corn)

1 Sauté or steam-fry the onion, garlic and peppers in the oil for 5 minutes, or until fairly soft.
2 For chicken fajitas, rub the seasoning into the chicken and grill until cooked. Mix into the vegetables. For bean fajitas, add the fajita seasoning to the vegetables during cooking, then stir in the beans and remove from the heat.
3 Spoon the salsa and/or guacamole into the middle of each tortilla and add the chicken or bean and vegetable mixture. Fold up and eat while they are still warm.

MAINTENANCE PHASE (PER PERSON) ✅
increase to 1 large tortilla

COOK'S NOTES
Storage instructions
eat straightaway
Allergy suitability
gluten, wheat (if you use corn tortillas) and dairy free
vegan (if you use beans rather than chicken)

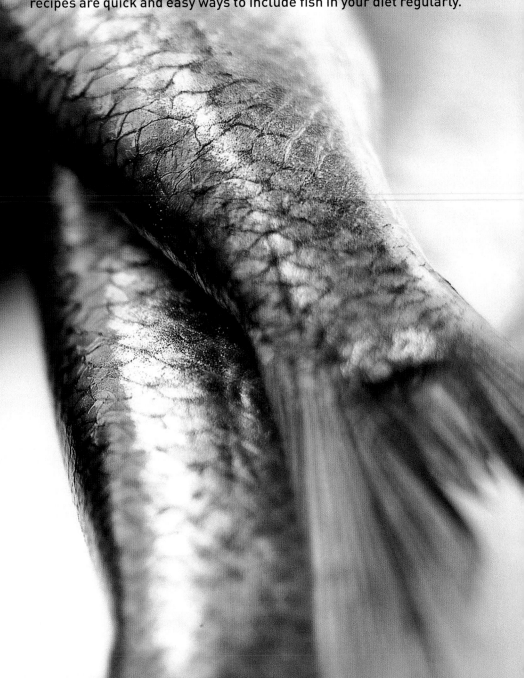

FISH

Not only is fish an excellent source of protein to help balance blood sugar but oily fish like salmon, trout and mackerel also provide omega-3 essential oils to aid heart, hormone, skin and brain function. These recipes are quick and easy ways to include fish in your diet regularly.

Pesto-baked salmon

Just two ingredients and 18 minutes in the oven produce a fabulous fish dish that is perfect for a quick supper with friends.

SERVES 2
2 salmon fillets
1 tbsp pesto

1 Preheat the oven to 180°C/350°F/Gas 4.
2 Place the salmon fillets on a baking tray or in a roasting tin and spread the pesto on top of each.
3 Bake for 18 minutes, or until the flesh flakes easily when pressed.

MAINTENANCE PHASE (PER PERSON) ✅
increase to 90g (3¼oz) (dry weight) quinoa. Or add 4–5 chopped sun-dried tomato pieces to the 65g (2¼oz) (dry weight) quinoa

COOK'S NOTES
Serving suggestion (per person)
65g (2¼oz) quinoa (dry weight) and steamed or roasted vegetables
Variations
use chicken instead of salmon fillets (cook at 190°C/375°F/Gas 5 for 25 minutes). Use tapenade instead of pesto
Storage instructions
better eaten fresh, but you could chill leftovers and eat the next day
Allergy suitability
gluten and wheat free

Hot-smoked fish with a lemon and caper dressing

Fillets of hot-smoked fish make brilliantly easy meals, as they are ready to eat and taste amazing. They are available in supermarkets and can be served simply with a salad and potatoes or beans.

SERVES 2
2 hot-smoked fish fillets (salmon, trout or mackerel, from supermarkets), about 75g–100g (2¾ – 3½oz) each

FOR THE DRESSING
1 tbsp lemon juice
2 tbsp extra virgin olive oil
1 tsp coarse-grain mustard
1 tbsp capers, well rinsed and drained (optional)
1 tbsp flat leaf parsley, finely chopped (optional)
Freshly ground black pepper
Pinch of salt or low-sodium salt (optional – the capers and mustard should provide enough salt on their own so check before adding)

Make the dressing by mixing all the ingredients together then pour over the fish and serving accompaniments (see Cook's Notes)

MAINTENANCE PHASE (PER PERSON) ✅
increase to 4 small baby new potatoes, or 90g (3¼oz) (dry weight) quinoa

COOK'S NOTES
Serving suggestion (per person)
with salad or steamed vegetables (such as courgettes and cauliflower, or broccoli or peas), and 3 small boiled baby new potatoes, 65g (2¼oz) (dry weight) quinoa or ½ x 410g (14½oz) can flageolet beans, rinsed and drained
Variations
use Dijon mustard instead of coarse-grain mustard, and vary the herbs and vegetables
Storage instructions
the fish and dressing can be chilled and eaten the next day
Allergy suitability
gluten, wheat and dairy free

Harissa-spiced tuna steak

Fresh tuna steak has a much meatier flavour and texture than other fish, which helps it to carry the strong flavours of the harissa spices. Sadly, it is not sensible to have tuna (or other carnivorous fish like swordfish or marlin) more than a couple of times a month as they have been shown to contain high levels of the harmful heavy metal mercury. Take particular care if you are pregnant.

COOK'S NOTES
Serving suggestion (per person)
½ x 410g (14½oz) can mixed pulses or butterbeans, or 65g (2¼oz) (dry weight) quinoa plus a large mixed salad
Variations
omit the harissa paste and simply season the tuna with black pepper and sea salt or low-sodium salt
Storage instructions
better eaten fresh, but you could chill leftovers and eat hot or cold the next day
Allergy suitability
gluten, wheat, dairy and yeast free

SERVES 2
2 tbsp harissa paste (from supermarkets)
1 tbsp lemon juice
2 tuna steaks (washed and dried on kitchen paper)
1 tsp oil, for frying

1 Mix the harissa with the lemon juice and spread over the tuna to coat thoroughly on all sides. Place in the fridge to marinate if time allows (ideally for 2 hours, but 10 minutes also makes a difference).
2 Heat the oil in a large frying pan and add both tuna steaks. Cook over a fairly high heat for 2–3 minutes then turn and cook on the other side. Fresh tuna can be eaten raw, so serve it as rare or as well done as you like.

MAINTENANCE PHASE (PER PERSON) ✅
add a large portion (as much as you like) of steamed green beans (or cooked green beans in a can or jar) or sugarsnap peas. Or increase the quinoa to 90g (3¼oz) (dry weight)

Puttanesca pasta with tuna

Pasta can be enjoyed on my diet: serve wholemeal pasta and include some form of protein in the sauce. Whereas white pasta is very high GL, wholemeal pasta is a lower GL option and allows you to eat far more.

COOK'S NOTES
Serving suggestion (per person)
a huge mixed salad, with plenty of cherry tomatoes, red onion, spinach, rocket and watercress
Variations
add wilted spinach or rocket. Replace puttanesca sauce with any other tomato-based pasta sauce. Use 75g (2¾oz) chicken goujons or 1 tbsp pine nuts (per person) in place of the tuna.
Allergy suitability
dairy free

SERVES 2
85g (3oz) wholemeal pasta
4 tbsp puttanesca sauce (ready-made tomato sauce for pasta, with capers, olives and anchovies)
185g (6½oz) can tuna, drained (140g (5oz) drained weight)

1 Cook the pasta according to the instructions on the packet, drain thoroughly then return to the pan.
2 Stir the sauce and the tuna through the pasta.

MAINTENANCE PHASE (PER PERSON) ✅
increase to 55g (2oz) pasta (dry weight)

Steamed salmon with stir-fried shiitake mushrooms

Shiitake mushrooms not only have a wonderfully smoky flavour and firm texture but they also contain special substances that have a powerful boosting effect on our immune system. If you cannot get hold of them, ordinary mushrooms also work well in this recipe.

SERVES 2
2 salmon fillets
2 tsp oil
150g (5¹/₂oz) pack shiitake mushrooms (or ordinary mushrooms), brushed or wiped clean with a dry piece of kitchen paper, and thickly sliced
Unlimited vegetables for stir-frying (try half a bag or about 200g (7oz) beansprouts, plus a sliced red pepper or handful of baby corn, or a couple of handfuls of baby or young leaf spinach or shredded spring greens)
1–2 tbsp tamari or soy sauce, to taste

1 Steam the salmon for 12–15 minutes, or until cooked (the fish should flake easily when pressed).
2 Meanwhile, heat the oil in a wok or frying pan (preferably one with a lid) and stir-fry the mushrooms for a few minutes, or until they soften and turn golden. Add the vegetables and tamari or soy sauce and turn down the heat to a gentle simmer. Cover the pan with a lid (or a couple of sheets of damp kitchen paper) to allow the vegetables to steam-fry.

MAINTENANCE PHASE (PER PERSON) ✔
increase the brown basmati rice to 65g or 95g (dry weight) quinoa

COOK'S NOTES
Serving suggestion (per person)
40g (1¹/₂oz) (dry weight) brown basmati rice or 65g (2¹/₄oz) (dry weight) quinoa
Variations
poach the salmon in place of steaming (in a pan of gently simmering water until cooked)
Storage instructions
not suitable for cooking in advance or reheating
Allergy suitability
gluten, wheat and dairy free (use tamari rather than soy sauce if you cannot eat wheat)

Peppers stuffed with smoked mackerel and beans

COOK'S NOTES
Serving suggestion (per person)
green salad
Variations
choose non-peppered smoked-
mackerel fillets for a milder
flavour. Add a chopped hard-boiled
egg for a kedgeree-style salad, or
use two hard-boiled eggs instead
of the fish for a vegetarian version
Allergy suitability
gluten, wheat and dairy free

As well as a strong flavour, peppered smoked mackerel fillets
add valuable omega-3 oils to this substantial stuffed-pepper dish.

SERVES 2
2 red peppers
2 peppered smoked mackerel fillets, about 75g (2³/₄oz)
     each, skinned, flaked and checked for bones
410g (14¹/₂oz) can cannellini beans, drained and rinsed
10cm (4in) chunk cucumber, diced
1 red onion, diced
1 handful cherry tomatoes, quartered or diced
6 Kalamata (or black) olives, pitted and halved

FOR THE DRESSING
1 tbsp olive oil
2 tsp lemon juice
Freshly ground black pepper

1 Preheat the oven to 200°C/400°F/Gas 6.
2 Cut the top off the peppers (reserving the lid), remove the seeds
and pith, and slice off the bulbous part inside the pepper that sits
below the stalk and contains most of the seeds.
3 Place the peppers upright on a baking tray and put the tops
back on. Roast for 25 minutes then drain off the water that will
have accumulated in the peppers.
4 While the peppers are cooking mix together the remaining
ingredients and stir in the dressing.
5 Fill the peppers with the mackerel salad and serve any remaining
salad alongside them.

MAINTENANCE PHASE (PER PERSON) ✔
add 3 small boiled baby new potatoes or 65g (2¹/₄oz) quinoa
(dry weight) to the salad mixture

King prawn pilaff

Seafood such as prawns is very low in fat and high in protein and minerals. Serving it with brown basmati rice, the lowest GL of all rice grains (because of its low starch content), makes this a low-GL but filling meal.

SERVES 2
1 tsp coconut oil or olive oil
1 red onion, thinly sliced or diced
1 red pepper, seeded and diced
10 cherry tomatoes, roughly chopped
$1/2$ tsp salt or low-sodium salt
90g (3$1/4$oz) brown basmati rice
200ml (7fl oz) boiling water
225g (8oz) cooked, peeled king prawns (or ordinary prawns)
2 drops hot pepper sauce (optional, or to taste)

1 Heat the oil in a pan and gently sauté the onion and pepper for 5 minutes, or until soft.
2 Add the tomatoes, salt and rice, and stir-fry for another minute or so.
3 Pour the water into the pan, bring up to the boil then cover and simmer gently for around 15–20 minutes, or until the rice is cooked.
4 Stir the prawns through the pilaff and add the hot pepper sauce to taste.

MAINTENANCE PHASE (PER PERSON) ✔
increase to 65g (2$1/4$oz) (dry weight) brown basmati rice

COOK'S NOTES
Serving suggestion (per person)
with a mixed salad or steamed vegetables
Variations
use a diced courgette instead of the pepper. Use a leek to replace the onion. Add a teaspoon of dried chilli flakes to give the dish extra kick
Storage instructions
best eaten freshly cooked
Allergy suitability
gluten, wheat and dairy free

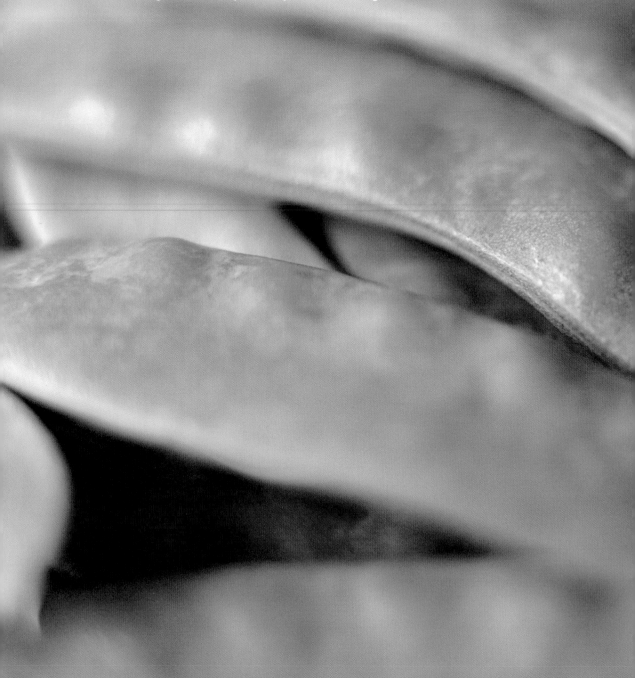

VEGETARIAN

So often vegetarian dishes lack imagination, resorting to cheese for protein. These recipes feature unusual and interesting ingredients to provide you with a range of nutrients and flavours.

Cashew and sesame quinoa

Quinoa looks and cooks like couscous but is in fact a fruit seed that contains complete protein and lots of minerals, making it ideal for vegetarians and vegans. This pilaf-like dish is unbelievably tasty and the raw veg provides more low-GL fibre and vitamins.

SERVES 2
140g (5oz) quinoa
1 tsp Marigold Reduced Salt Vegetable Bouillon powder
3–4 tbsp fresh or frozen and thawed petits pois or peas
2 tbsp cashew nuts
2 tsp sesame oil
1 tbsp tamari or soy sauce
2 tsp lemon juice
1 carrot, julienned (finely sliced lengthways into matchsticks)
6 spring onions, finely sliced on the diagonal
Freshly ground black pepper

1 Add the quinoa and bouillon powder to a saucepan, cover with double the amount of cold water and bring to the boil. Cover and simmer for 13 minutes, or until all the water has been absorbed and the quinoa grains are soft and fluffy.

2 Add the peas and stir through for a couple of minutes then remove from the heat. They will cook or soften slightly in the residual warmth.

3 Combine with the remaining ingredients, tossing thoroughly to mix all the flavours and allow the quinoa to absorb the liquid seasonings.

MAINTENANCE PHASE (PER PERSON) ●
have a 5 GL dessert such as a piece of fruit or marzipan truffles (see page 140) afterwards (see pages 138–142 for more dessert ideas)

COOK'S NOTES
Serving suggestion (per person)
on its own or with salad
Variations
omit the cashew nuts if you have a nut allergy – the quinoa provides complete protein on its own. Serve with a piece of grilled chicken or fish, if you like
Storage instructions
keep chilled for up to 3 days
Allergy suitability
gluten, wheat and dairy free (use tamari instead of soy sauce if you cannot eat wheat)
vegan

Chestnut and butterbean soup

This is fast, easy and deliciously filling. One of the most popular dishes at the Holford 100% Health Workshops and from *The Holford Low-GL Diet Cookbook*.

SERVES 2

200g (7oz) cooked and peeled chestnuts (available vacuum-packed in boxes, cans or jars)
410g (14¹/₂oz) can of butterbeans, rinsed and drained
1 medium white onion, chopped
1 large carrot, peeled and chopped
3 tsp Marigold Reduced Salt Vegetable Bouillon powder dissolved in 600ml (1 pint) water
Freshly ground black pepper

1 Place all the ingredients (except for a handful of the chestnuts and the pepper) in a saucepan. Cover with a lid and bring to the boil. Simmer gently for 15–20 minutes, or until tender.
2 Purée the soup in a blender or food processor until smooth, and season with the black pepper.
3 Sprinkle the reserved chestnuts on top.

MAINTENANCE PHASE (PER PERSON) ●
have 1 rough oatcake with the soup

COOK'S NOTES
Storage instructions
keep chilled for no more than 4 days
Allergy suitability
gluten, wheat, dairy and yeast free
vegan

Warm tomato and olive mixed-pulse salad

A strongly flavoured vegan-friendly dish that can be served hot or cold.

SERVES 2
1 tsp olive oil
1 red onion, diced
410g (14¹/₂oz) can mixed pulses, drained and rinsed
2 tbsp of good quality tomato-based pasta sauce or 1 tbsp sun-dried tomato paste or pesto
2 tbsp black olives, pitted and roughly chopped
Freshly ground black pepper, to taste

1 Heat the oil in a saucepan and gently fry the onion for about 2 minutes.
2 Add the remaining ingredients and stir.

MAINTENANCE PHASE (PER PERSON) ●
increase to 70g (2¹/₂oz) quinoa (dry weight)

COOK'S NOTES
Serving suggestion (per person)
35g (1¹/₄oz) quinoa (half a large serving) (dry weight) and a large green salad, or with a chicken breast or fish fillet and salad
Variations
omit the olives if you prefer – you could add some strips of roasted pepper instead. Also delicious cold
Storage instructions
keeps well in the fridge for up to 4 days
Allergy suitability
gluten, wheat and dairy free
vegan

Creamy mushrooms on polenta slices

Pre-cooked polenta (cornmeal cooked to form a hard block that can be sliced up and grilled) is a brilliant time-saver. Buy it in plastic-wrapped blocks from supermarkets (it should be in the rice and pasta sections) ready for an almost instant meal.

SERVES 2
250g (9oz) precooked polenta, sliced about 1cm (1/2in) thick
2 tsp coconut oil or olive oil
225g (8oz) mushrooms, sliced
2 tsp Marigold Reduced Salt Vegetable Bouillon powder
6 tbsp boiling water
2 tbsp tahini

1 Preheat the grill to a medium-high.
2 Grill the polenta slices for 5–10 minutes, or until they start to turn golden.
3 Meanwhile, heat the oil in a frying pan and sauté the mushrooms gently for a few minutes, or until cooked.
4 Stir the bouillon powder and water into the tahini, mixing well.
5 Add the tahini mixture to the pan of mushrooms and stir for a few minutes while it simmers until it becomes thick and creamy.
6 Place the polenta slices on plates and spoon the creamy mushroom mixture on top.

MAINTENANCE PHASE (PER PERSON) ✔
stir 1/2 x 410g (14 1/2oz) can of cannellini, butter or borlotti beans through the mushrooms, or increase the polenta to 200g (7oz)

COOK'S NOTES
Serving suggestion (per person)
mixed salad
Variations
pan-fry the polenta slices in a little oil for a few minutes each side to pick up some colour and crispen the outside slightly. Top the polenta with wilted spinach and 2 poached eggs. Use one slice toasted pumpernickel-style rye bread instead of the polenta
Allergy suitability
gluten, wheat, dairy and yeast free
vegan

Soy and sesame tofu steam-fry

For any tofuphobes out there, forget your prejudices and try this Chinese-inspired dish – smoked tofu is a much meatier and firmer texture than bland, plain tofu, and the rich soy and sesame dressing adds lots of flavour.

COOK'S NOTES
Serving suggestion (per person)
serve the tofu and vegetables with 40g (1¹/₂oz) (dry weight) brown basmati rice or 65g (2¹/₄oz) (dry weight) quinoa – drizzle any remaining dressing from the steam-fry over the top
Variations
use different vegetables for steam-frying (such as broccoli, tenderstem, sliced peppers, baby corn, mange tout or beansprouts)
Storage instructions
best eaten fresh
Allergy suitability
gluten and dairy free (if using tamari – wheat-free soy sauce) vegan

SERVES 2
1 tbsp coconut oil or olive oil
200g (7oz) smoked tofu, drained on kitchen paper and cut into cubes (the best-tasting tofu is the flavoured varieties such as sesame, almond or herb tofu, from health-food stores. Plain smoked tofu can be found in most supermarkets, however)
About 1 tbsp tamari or soy sauce
1 tbsp lemon juice
1 tbsp toasted sesame oil
Unlimited vegetables for steam-frying (such as beansprouts, peppers, onions, baby corn, spring greens or pak choi – buy a bag of ready-prepared vegetables for stir-frying to save time)
1 tbsp tamari, or soy sauce or water (for the steam-fry)

1 Heat the oil in a wok or frying pan and stir-fry the tofu for a few minutes, or until it turns golden on all sides. Remove from the wok or pan.
2 Mix 1 tbsp tamari or soy sauce with the lemon juice and sesame oil, and pour over the tofu. Set to one side to keep warm while you steam-fry the vegetables.
3 Add the vegetables to the wok or pan and stir-fry for a minute or so. Add 1 tbsp water, soy sauce or tamari and cover to allow the vegetables to steam for a couple of minutes, or until cooked (checking halfway to make sure the pan hasn't boiled dry – you can always add a splash more liquid). If you don't have a lid you can improvise by soaking a couple of sheets of kitchen paper in cold water and placing them over the food in the wok to cover it, allowing the water to create moisture in the pan.

MAINTENANCE PHASE (PER PERSON) ✅
increase to 65g (2¹/₄oz) (dry weight) brown basmati rice or 90g (3¹/₄oz) (dry weight) quinoa

Rice and vegetables with a tahini sauce

The creamy sauce from tahini (sesame paste) turns ordinary basmati rice into a risotto-style dish without the need for using starchy, high-GL risotto rice or to add cream or butter. It is also surprisingly filling and warming if you are in need of comfort food.

SERVES 2
90g (3¹/₄oz) brown basmati rice
1 tsp Marigold Reduced Salt Vegetable Bouillon powder
1 tsp coconut oil or olive oil
1 onion, diced
1 garlic clove, crushed (optional)

FOR THE SAUCE
1–2 tsp Marigold Reduced Salt Vegetable Bouillon powder
Around 6 tbsp boiling water
2 tbsp tahini
2 tbsp fresh flat leaf parsley leaves, finely chopped (optional)

1 Pour plenty of boiling water into a pan and add the rice. Add the bouillon powder and bring to the boil. Cover and simmer gently for 15–20 minutes, or until the rice is cooked. Drain and keep warm.
2 Meanwhile, heat the oil in a pan and sauté the onion and garlic, if using, for about 2 minutes, or until soft.
3 To make the sauce, stir the bouillon powder and boiling water into the tahini until it forms a smooth, creamy sauce (it will curdle at the beginning, but keep stirring and it will come together). Check the seasoning and add more water if the flavour is too strong. Stir in the parsley, if using.
4 Stir the onion and garlic, and the sauce, into the cooked rice.

MAINTENANCE PHASE (PER PERSON) ✔
increase to 65g (2¹/₄oz) (dry weight) brown basmati rice

COOK'S NOTES
Serving suggestion (per person)
with steamed vegetables, such as broccoli, sugarsnap peas, mange tout or asparagus
Variations
use a leek instead of onion. Meat eaters could stir in 2 tbsp cooked, peeled prawns, flaked tuna or sliced chicken, turkey or lean ham
Storage instructions
best eaten fresh
Allergy suitability
gluten, wheat, dairy and yeast free vegan

Grilled goat's cheese salad with roasted peppers and walnuts

The simple flavour combination of goat's cheese, roasted peppers and walnuts is very successful, and the salty, creamy goat's cheese is just heavenly when it is warm and oozing over the salad.

SERVES 2

2 round slices of firm goat's cheese, about 75–100g (2¹/₂–3¹/₂oz) each
4 tbsp roasted peppers in oil, drained and oil reserved for the dressing (available in jars or fresh from the deli), roughly chopped
2 tbsp roughly chopped walnuts (if time, you could lightly toast these in a dry frying pan until just turning golden)
1 bag, about 150g (5¹/₂oz) fully prepared mixed salad leaves, organic where possible
Freshly ground black pepper

1 Place the goat's cheese on foil and grill under a medium heat for approximately 5 minutes, or until golden, bubbling on top and starting to ooze.
2 Meanwhile, construct the salad by tossing the peppers and walnuts through the salad leaves and then placing on serving plates.
3 When the goat's cheese is ready, carefully lift it off the foil with a spatula and spoon one into the middle of each plate. Season with plenty of black pepper and drizzle with up to 1 tbsp of the marinating oil from the peppers over each plate.

MAINTENANCE PHASE (PER PERSON) ✔
increase to 90g (3¹/₄oz) (dry weight) quinoa or 4 boiled baby new potatoes

COOK'S NOTES
Serving suggestion (per person)
with 65g (2¹/₄oz) (dry weight) quinoa or 3 boiled baby new potatoes
Variations
replace the peppers with marinated mushrooms or artichoke hearts, or mixed vegetable antipasti. Replace walnuts with pine nuts. Dress with balsamic vinegar as well as/instead of the marinating oil if you prefer
Storage instructions
eat while the goat's cheese is still warm
Allergy suitability
gluten and wheat free
vegetarian

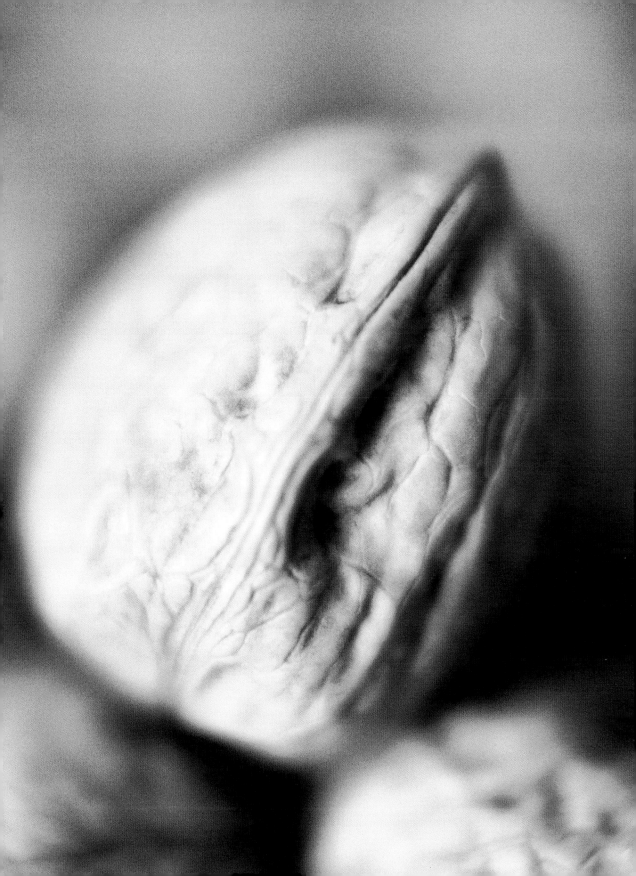

EASY DESSERTS

The following recipes all contain 5⒢⒧, so that they are suitable for the occasional dessert during the weight-loss phase (1–2 times a week from week two onwards, as part of the 45⒢⒧ per day total so they could replace the 5⒢⒧ quota allocated for drinks), or they can also be eaten as 5 GL snacks. They also all include adaptations to increase the serving size to 10⒢⒧ so that they can be enjoyed as more substantial desserts during the maintenance phase, when you are allowed more ⒢⒧ per day.

Low-GL pudding tips

⟶ Have no more than 5⒢⒧ for drinks and desserts combined (or 10⒢⒧ on the maintenance diet).

⟶ Limit saturated fat and avoid cream and full-fat cheeses.

⟶ As a general guide, fruit- and protein-based puddings (the ones that contain eggs, dairy products or nuts) such as fruit fools, cheesecakes, egg custards or mousses and nutty biscuits will have lower ⒢⒧ than sugar- and carbohydrate-based options such as wheat biscuits, chocolate cake and syrupy flapjacks.

⟶ The low-GL diet moves away from the idea of desserts as 'treats'. If you need to treat yourself, choose a good-health option such as a massage, fresh flowers or meeting up with a friend instead.

Chocolate-covered nuts

You can buy these, but they tend to use lots of cheap, sugary chocolate. If you make your own you can use just a little dark chocolate that is high in cocoa solids (at least 70 per cent) and low in sugar. The protein from the nuts helps to lower the GL naturally as well.

SERVES 2
15g (1/2oz) good-quality dark chocolate, broken into pieces
25g (1oz) shelled mixed nuts, such as almonds, macadamia nuts, hazelnuts, Brazil nuts or cashew nuts

1 Line a baking tray with baking parchment.
2 Gently melt the chocolate (either in a microwave or in a heatproof bowl over a pan of hot water).
3 Tip the nuts into the melted chocolate and stir to coat. Spoon onto the baking tray and chill for at least 15–20 minutes, or until set.
4 Divide into two portions.

MAINTENANCE PHASE (PER PERSON) ✓
double up the quantities

COOK'S NOTES
Variations
use desiccated coconut for some of the nut mix
Storage instructions
keeps for up to 1 month. Best kept in an airtight container in a cool, dry place
Allergy suitability
gluten, wheat and dairy free (choose dairy-free chocolate)
vegan (depending on the chocolate)

Chocolate

If you have no time to prepare a snack from scratch, or are eating out and want to round off a meal with something sweet, a square or two of good-quality dark chocolate is still allowed. Dark chocolate contains more antioxidants, and brands with a high cocoa-solid content (at least 70 per cent) contain less sugar than cheaper ones, which rely on sugar for flavour.

SERVES 1
10g (1/4oz) chocolate (buy a small bar to limit temptation)

MAINTENANCE PHASE (PER PERSON) ✓
double up the quantities for a 10 GL treat

COOK'S NOTES
Allergy suitability
gluten, wheat and dairy free (choose dairy-free dark chocolate)
vegan (if you have dairy-free dark chocolate)

Marzipan truffles

Allergy suitability
gluten, wheat, dairy and yeast free
vegetarian

Health note
Because this recipe contains
raw eggs always choose organic
or free range eggs to reduce
the likelihood of salmonella
contamination, and do not serve
to young children, pregnant
women, the elderly or anyone
with a compromised immune
system.

This recipe is ideal for anyone with a sweet tooth, but is in fact very
low-GL, as the nuts and eggs provide plenty of protein while low-GL
xylitol replaces normal sugar. It first appeared in *The Holford Low-GL
Diet Cookbook* and we wanted to include it here as it can be mixed
together in minutes.

SERVES 2 (MAKES 8–10 TRUFFLES)
125g (4¹/₂oz) ground almonds
4 drops almond extract
1–2 tbsp xylitol
4 organic, free range egg yolks (or 3 egg yolks and 1 whole egg)
1 heaped tbsp finely chopped almonds

1 Mix the ground almonds, almond extract, xylitol and egg yolks
together until they form a smooth paste. Taste and adjust the
sweetness if necessary.
2 Shape into walnut-sized balls and roll each ball in a saucer
of the finely chopped almonds until the outside is coated in nuts.
3 Place on a plate and store in the fridge until firm.

MAINTENANCE PHASE (PER PERSON) ✔
for a 10 GL dessert, melt a few squares of dark chocolate, about
40g (1¹/₂oz), in a heatproof bowl over a pan of hot water and dip
in the truffles to coat before sprinkling with the chopped almonds.
Chill to let the chocolate harden (discard any excess chocolate
before temptation strikes and you find yourself licking the bowl)

Tip Keep the leftover egg whites in the fridge and add to omelettes
or scrambled eggs (the egg whites are very high in protein and low
in fat, and they help make very light and fluffy egg dishes).

Yogurt and fresh fruit

If you are at home and have more time, you can make more of this simple dessert by slicing the fruit and placing it in the base of a glass or bowl, then spoon on the yogurt and scatter toasted flaked almonds on top.

SERVES 2
1 small–medium apple or pear, cored and diced, or 4 plums
   or apricots, stoned and diced
150g (5¹/₂oz) blueberries, or other berries, rinsed
300g (11oz) live natural yogurt or soya yogurt

Toss all the fruit together and serve with the yogurt.

MAINTENANCE PHASE (PER PERSON)
for a 10 GL dessert, add more fruit (such as a kiwi fruit, a small banana or an orange, peach or nectarine)

COOK'S NOTES
Variations
use frozen mixed berries when fresh berries are out of season (defrost and sweeten with a little xylitol if they are too tart)
Storage instructions
best eaten the same day. If not eating immediately, drizzle the fruit with lemon juice to prevent discolouration, cover and chill. Add the yogurt when ready to serve
Allergy suitability
gluten, wheat and dairy free (if using soya yogurt) vegetarian (or vegan if using soya yogurt)

Raspberries with sweet tahini sauce

Reminiscent of the messes made with ice cream and mashed strawberries by children, this is not the most elegant of desserts, but the sweetened tahini has a fudge-like flavour and mixes with the soft fruit to create a luscious, pink mixture that is simply delicious. It is also very low-GL and high in bone-strengthening minerals.

SERVES 2
2 tbsp tahini
4 tbsp water
About 2 tbsp xylitol, to taste (some brands of tahini are more
   bitter than others and may need more sweetening)
2 punnets raspberries, about 300g (10¹/₂oz) in total, rinsed

1 Mix the tahini with the water until it forms a smooth, creamy sauce (it will curdle at the beginning, but keep stirring and it will come together). Stir in the xylitol and adjust taste to check the sweetness.
2 Stir the raspberries into the sauce and spoon into two bowls.

MAINTENANCE PHASE (PER PERSON) ✔
for a 10 GL dessert, stir 4 tbsp whole rolled oats into the mixture

COOK'S NOTES
Variations
use chopped strawberries or other berries (or use frozen mixed summer fruits if berries are out of season). Replace tahini with unsalted hazelnut butter (from good health food stores)
Storage instructions
keep in the fridge for up to 2 days (bring up to room temperature and stir before serving, if the mixture separates)
Allergy suitability
gluten, wheat, dairy and yeast free (omit the oats from the maintenance phase)
vegan

Cereal bar

While many cereal bars or flapjacks are full of high-GL ingredients such as sugar, syrup, honey, brown rice syrup, dried fruit and puffed grains like corn or rice, there are increasing numbers of low-GL products on the market to look out for.

COOK'S NOTES
Allergy suitability
wheat and dairy free (check label on different brands)
vegan (depending on the brand)

SERVES 1
Fruitus bar (by Lyme Regis Foods, from supermarkets and health food stores), or other low-GL cereal bar (check that it doesn't have hidden sugars, as listed above)

MAINTENANCE PHASE (PER PERSON) ✅
have a 5 GL piece of fruit such as an apple afterwards

Ten-minute fruit crumble

This crumble is made on the hob in minutes. The nuts add protein to lower the sugar release from the carbohydrate and the GL score.

COOK'S NOTES
Variations
vary the nuts and seeds in the crumble (use half almonds and half roughly chopped hazelnuts or pecans)
Storage instructions
best eaten warm but it can also be eaten cold, or kept in the fridge for up to 2 days and reheated gently (in the microwave or just tip the mixture into a pan and heat it all up)
Allergy suitability
wheat, dairy and yeast free
vegan

SERVES 2
3 plums or apricots, or 1 large pear or a small cooking apple, or 100g (3½oz) trimmed rhubarb, washed and cut into chunks
Splash of water
A little xylitol to sweeten to taste, if necessary (you will need around 2 tbsp for the rhubarb, but only 1–2 tsp for the other fruits)

FOR THE CRUMBLE
1 tbsp coconut oil or olive oil
1 tbsp xylitol
50g (1¾oz) whole oat flakes
4 tbsp ground almonds

1 Place the fruit in a saucepan with the water, cover and stew gently until the fruit softens, stirring from time to time. Taste and sweeten with xylitol if necessary.
2 Meanwhile, make the crumble. Gently heat the oil in a frying pan with the xylitol, add the oats and toast them for around 3 minutes, or until they start to colour and crisp slightly.
3 Stir in the almonds and remove from the heat.
4 Spoon the stewed fruit into small bowls and cover with the crumble.

MAINTENANCE PHASE (PER PERSON) ✅
increase the fruit filling to 4 plums or apricots, 2 pears or 1 large cooking apple, or 200g (7oz) rhubarb, and increase the oats to 75g (2¾oz) (you may need to add a little extra xylitol to sweeten)

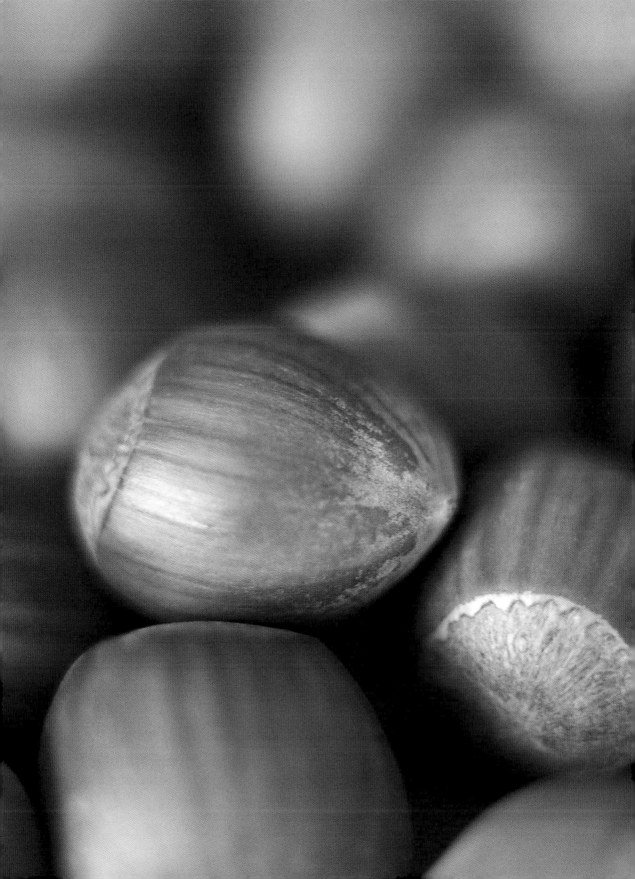

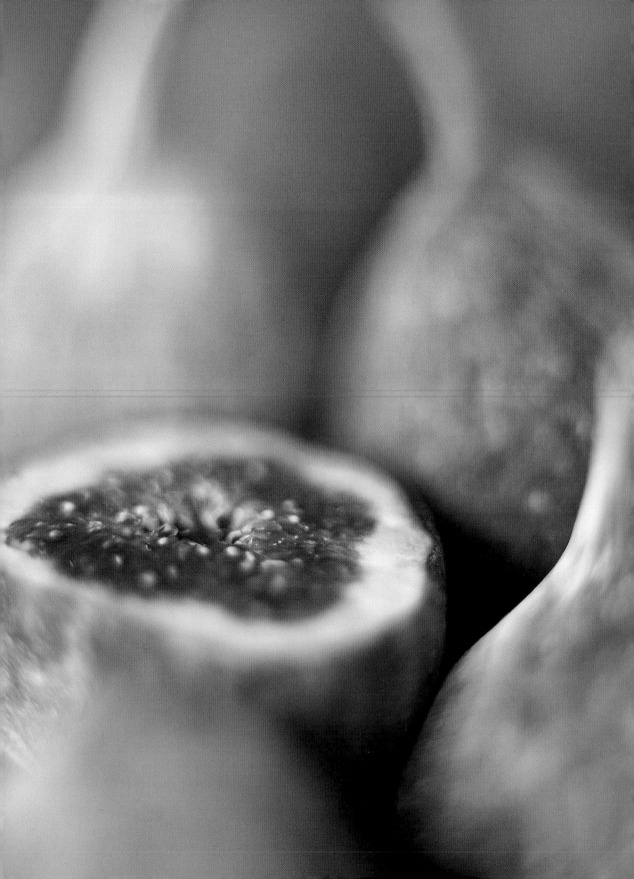

8 EATING OUT ON THE HOLFORD LOW-GL DIET

'Eating out' can mean anything from grabbing a quick takeaway to enjoying a three-course meal in a restaurant, or a lunchtime snack and a cappuccino in a sandwich bar. This section concentrates mainly on common takeaway foods and casual eating because that is the area where we are likely to be the most impulsive and the least prepared.

Remember – just because you paid for it, or because it is put on the table, it doesn't mean you have to eat it.

Top tips
→ Don't accept a piece of bread before your meal arrives (your 7 GL carbohydrate quota will have gone before you have even started!) Ask for a bowl of olives instead.
→ If you aren't particularly tempted by any of the puddings on offer, don't have one!
→ If everyone else is choosing starters and there are no healthy options available, ask for a mixed salad instead (with the dressing on the side).

Many restaurants are able to cater for special dietary needs if they are given some advance warning. So if you are booking ahead it is worth explaining your needs in advance. For healthy lunchtime alternatives to shop-bought temptations, see the Food on the Move section starting on page 98.

This section is not intended to ruin your fun, but is designed to help you to stay close to the low-GL guidelines and avoid undoing all your hard work. Different options and advice follows, according to the different types of cuisine you might want to eat.

FRENCH

Low-GL friendly:

→ Olives are a healthier option than bread.

→ Choose salade niçoise.

→ Choose mussels (moules).

→ Combine meat, fish or seafood with plenty of salad or vegetables and 3 small potatoes or 2 tbsp beans or lentils.

Foods to avoid:

→ Creamy, cheesy sauces.

→ Fatty, sugary pastries.

ITALIAN

Low-GL friendly:

→ Olives rather than bread or breadsticks to nibble on.

→ Carpaccio.

→ Melon with Parma ham (remove the fatty rind if possible).

→ Artichoke.

→ Grilled meat, fish and seafood with salads and vegetables. Antipasti platters (go for vegetable antipasti where possible).

→ Choose a thin-based pizza and share with someone. Opt for vegetable and lean meat (such as chicken or fish) toppings.

→ Tomato sauces.

Foods to avoid:

→ Risottos, pasta and gnocchi dishes.

→ Cream or cheese-based sauces, including mozzarella.

SPANISH/TAPAS

Ask for your meal to be prepared with less oil, as Spanish food is often drenched in olive oil.

Low-GL friendly:

→ Olives are a better choice than bread or breadsticks to nibble on.

→ Choose vegetable dishes.

→ Choose Spanish omelette.

→ Remove the fatty rind from meats such as Serrano ham.

Foods to avoid:

⇢ Avoid fatty meats and sausages like chorizo.

GREEK AND TURKISH

Low-GL friendly:

⇢ Fill up on salads like Greek salad, and grilled fish.

⇢ Have plenty of salad in your kebab.

⇢ Kebabs are fine as long as the meat is lean and the kebabs are served with vegetables.

Foods to avoid:

⇢ Oily dishes, such as moussaka.

⇢ Fatty cuts of meat (such as in lamb kebabs).

⇢ Limit your portion of white (high-GL) rice to 1 tbsp.

⇢ Very sweet pastries.

MEXICAN

Low-GL friendly:

⇢ Fajitas (have just 1 fajita wrap and avoid the sour cream and cheese – fill up on salad, vegetables and chicken or beans, salsa and guacamole).

Foods to avoid:

⇢ Soured cream and cheese fillings for fajitas and burritos.

THAI AND CHINESE

Low-GL friendly:

⇢ Broths.

⇢ Salads.

⇢ Meat, fish and vegetable stir-fries.

⇢ Limit yourself to 1 tbsp rice.

Foods to avoid:

⇢ Dishes where noodles or rice are integral to the dish such as pad thai or stir-fried rice, as the portion sizes greatly exceed the 7 GL limits.

⇢ Sweet chilli dipping sauce, which is high in sugar.

⇢ High-fat satay sauce.

⇢ Avoid sugar-based sweet-and-sour sauces.

JAPANESE
Low-GL friendly:
⇢ Miso soup and broths.
⇢ Salads.
⇢ Sashimi and sushi contain excellent protein but the sticky white rice on sushi greatly adds to the GL, so limit the amount you eat.

Foods to avoid:
⇢ Sweet-and-sour dishes and sugar-based sauces, such as teriyaki and sweet chilli dipping sauce.
⇢ Fried dishes such as tempura.

INDIAN
Low-GL friendly:
⇢ Tandoori dishes are the best choice.
⇢ Sag channa (spinach with chickpeas).
⇢ Lentil dhal.
⇢ Choose wholemeal chapatti instead of white rice or naan bread.
⇢ Curried vegetables are likely to include potatoes, and so should be counted as your carbohydrate serving instead of rice or chapatti.
⇢ Tomato-based sauces like Madras are a better option than creamy sauces.

Foods to avoid:
⇢ Ghee- (butter-) drenched curried sauces.
⇢ Creamy sauces such as masala.
⇢ Sugary mango chutney – pickles (like lime pickle) contain less sugar.

AMERICAN/BURGER BAR
Low-GL friendly:
⇢ Choose a lean beefburger with half the bun or half a small baked potato.
⇢ Have a side salad to accompany the meal (not mayonnaise-laden coleslaw).

Foods to avoid:
⇢ Avoid sugary ketchup – go for tomato salsa instead.
⇢ American-style thin-cut French fries.

Fish and chips

As they are such a firm takeaway favourite, fish and chips need a special mention. They are always bad news because of the saturated fat content and the high cooking temperatures, but, if possible, opt for grilled fish without batter. Choose thick-cut chips if you must, as these have less surface area to absorb oil. Any more than 3 chips will take you well over your GL allowance. Choosing a side salad or mushy peas will help you fill up in a more healthy way.

DESSERTS

Almost all restaurant desserts are likely to be very high GL, but, if you can't resist, limit the damage by choosing something that contains protein and is low in carbohydrate – such as a scoop of ice cream, or fruit with crème fraîche, and either share your portion or leave some of it.

CHEESE PLATTER

Choose soft cheeses like Brie and soft goat's cheese, which are lower in saturated fat than hard cheeses like Cheddar and Parmesan. Have a small amount of a mature cheese for maximum flavour without having to eat a lot. Choose oatcakes rather than crackers or wheat biscuits, and have plenty of celery instead of high-GL grapes.

No foods are banned on the low-GL diet, but by being more food-aware and planning ahead you can enjoy the flavours of different styles of cuisine and the pleasure of eating out in any situation without worry. You can be confident that by following these guidelines and by watching your portion size you won't upset your blood sugar levels or gain unnecessary weight. When in doubt, just keep to the made easy rules in Chapter 3 and don't feel guilty about having the odd dessert now and again.

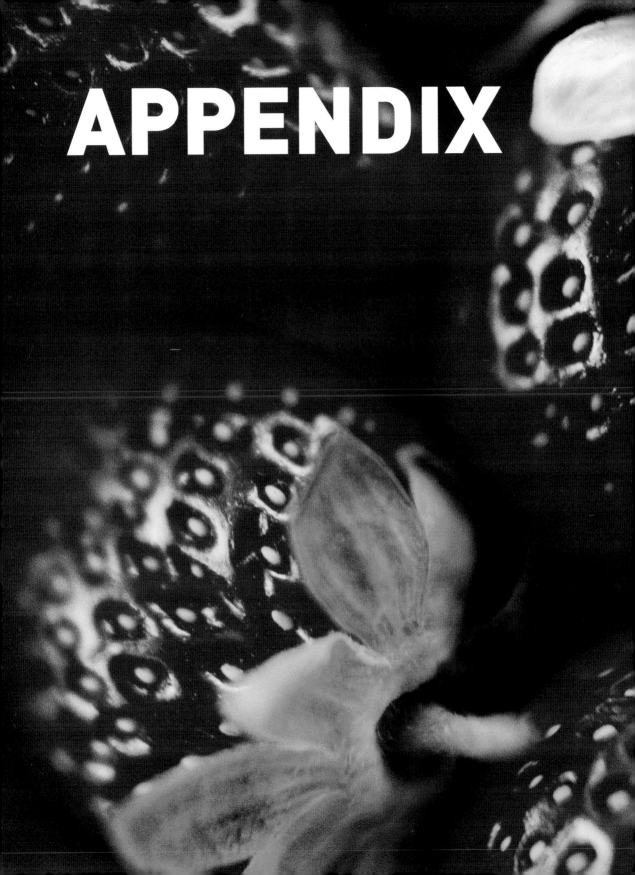

APPENDIX

GUIDE TO ABBREVIATIONS AND MEASURES

British (imperial)	Metric
1oz	28g
2oz	55g
3oz	85g
4oz	115g
5oz	140g
6oz	175g
7oz	200g
8oz	225g

Teaspoon and tablespoon measurements are used throughout the book.

1 teaspoon (tsp) = 5ml
1 tablespoon (tbsp) = 15ml
(**Note** Australian tablespoons are 20ml)

US cup measurements for liquids
250ml/9fl oz = 1 cup, 125ml (4fl oz) = ½ cup

VITAMINS
Most vitamins are measured in milligrams or micrograms. Vitamins A, D and E used to be measured in International Units (iu), a measurement designed to standardise the various forms of these vitamins, which have different potencies.

1 gram (g) = 1,000 milligrams (mg) = 1,000,000 micrograms (mcg, also written µg)

DAILY SUPPLEMENTS – GUIDELINES

Vitamins	Optimum daily intake	Health benefits
Vitamin A	1,500mcg	improves skin and immunity
Vitamin B1 (thiamine)	25mg	makes energy
Vitamin B2 (riboflavin)	25mg	makes energy
Vitamin B3 (niacin)	50mg	lowers cholesterol
Vitamin B5 (pantothenate)	50mg	improves memory
vitamin B6 (pyridoxine)	50mg	balances hormones
Vitamin B12 (cobalamin)	10mcg	vital for energy
Folic acid	200mcg	protects your DNA
Biotin	50mcg	vital for children
Vitamin C	1,000mg	boosts immunity
Vitamin D	5mcg	builds bones
Vitamin E (d-alpha tocopherol)	100mg	protects arteries

Minerals	Optimum daily intake	Health benefits
Calcium	200mg	builds bones
Magnesium	150mg	keeps you relaxed
Iron	10mg	carries oxygen
Zinc	10mg	boosts immunity
Manganese	3mg	anti-ageing oxidant
Chromium	30mcg	balances blood sugar

Supplement: Hydroxycitric acid (HCA)
Daily intake: 900mg. Works best before meals. One 450mg tablet or capsule twice daily, 30 minutes before lunch and evening meal.
Health benefits: turns food into energy, not fat

Supplement: Chromium
Daily intake: 200-400mcg. 200 mcg taken twice daily, with midmorning and afternoon snacks
Health benefits: reduces sugar craving

Supplement: 5-hydroxytryptophan (5-HTP)
Daily intake: 100-200mg. 50mg taken with carbohydrate (such as fruit) twice daily, with midmorning and afternoon snacks
Health benefits: reduces sugar craving, improves mood

A word of caution: Don't take 5-HTP if you are on serotonin-re-uptake inhibitor drugs (SSRIs), such as Prozac, Xeroxat, Paroxetine or Lustral. Theoretically, taking both could overload you with serotonin. Although I know of no case as such, I don't recommend taking both antidepressant drugs and 5-HTP.

WEIGHT–HEIGHT CHART

The following charts show your ideal weight range for your height. If you're within your ideal weight range please don't aim to lose more than 4lb (2kg) a month.
If you are above the ideal weight range your target weight loss should be no more than 8lb (4kg) a month.

Women aged 25 and over

Height		Weight		
Feet	Metres	Lb	Stone/lb	Kg
4' 8"	1.42m	92–107lb	6st 8lb–7st 9lb	42–49kg
4' 9"	1.45m	94–110lb	6st 10lb–7st 12lb	43–50kg
4' 10"	1.47m	96–113lb	6st 12lb–8st 1lb	44–51kg
4' 11"	1.50m	99–116lb	7st 1lb–8st 4lb	45–53kg
5' 0"	1.52m	102–119lb	7st 4lb–8st 7lb	46–54kg
5' 1"	1.55m	105–122lb	7st 7lb–8st 10lb	48–55kg
5' 2"	1.57m	108–126lb	7st 10lb–9st	49–57kg
5' 3"	1.60m	111–130lb	7st 13lb–9st 4lb	50–59kg
5' 4"	1.63m	114–135lb	8st 2lb–9st 9lb	52–61kg
5' 5"	1.65m	118–139lb	8st 6lb–9st 13lb	54–63kg
5' 6"	1.68m	122–143lb	8st 10lb–10st 3lb	55–65kg
5' 7"	1.70m	126–147lb	9st–10st 7lb	57–67kg
5' 8"	1.73m	130–151lb	9st 4lb–10st 11lb	59–68kg
5' 9"	1.75m	134–155lb	9st 8lb–11st 1lb	61–70kg
5' 10"	1.78m	138–159lb	9st 12lb–11st 5lb	63–72kg

Men aged 25 and over

Height		Weight		
Feet	Metres	Lb	Stone/lb	Kg
5' 1"	1.55m	112–129lb	8–9st 3lb	51–59kg
5' 2"	1.57m	115–133lb	8st 3lb–9st 7lb	52–60kg
5' 3"	1.6m	118–136lb	8st 6lb–9st 10lb	54–62kg
5' 4"	1.63m	121–139lb	8st 9lb–9st 13lb	55–63kg
5' 5"	1.65m	124–143lb	8st 12lb–10st 3lb	56–65kg
5' 6"	1.68m	128–147lb	9st 2lb–10st 7lb	58–67kg
5' 7"	1.70m	132–152lb	9st 6lb–10st 12lb	60–69kg
5' 8"	1.73m	136–156lb	9st 10lb–11st 2lb	62–71kg
5' 9"	1.75m	140–160lb	10st–11st 6lb	64–73kg
5' 10"	1.78m	144–165lb	10st 4lb–11st 11lb	65–75kg
5' 11"	1.80m	148–170lb	10st 8lb–12st 2lb	67–77kg
6' 0"	1.83m	152–175lb	10st 12lb–12st 7lb	69–79kg
6' 1"	1.85m	156–180lb	11st 2lb–12st 12lb	71–82kg
6' 2"	1.88m	160–185lb	11st 6lb–13st 3lb	73–84kg
6' 3"	1.90m	164–190lb	11st 10lb–13st 8lb	74–86kg

FURTHER RESOURCES

Institute for Optimum Nutrition (ION)
ION runs the Homestudy Course and the three-year Nutrition Therapists'
Foundation Degree course. For details on courses, consultations and publications
send a stamped, addressed envelope to ION, Avalon House, 72 Lower Mortlake
Road, Richmond TW9 2JY. Tel: +44 (0)20 8614 7800.

Nutrition consultations
For a personal referral to a nutritional therapist in your area, visit
www.patrickholford.com and select the 'Advice' tab followed by 'Find a nutritionist'
for an immediate online referral. This service gives details on whom to see in the
UK. If there is no one available nearby, you can always do an online assessment –
see below.

Nutrition assessment online
You can have your own personal health and nutrition assessment online using my
100% Health questionnaire. This gives you a personalised assessment of your
current health, and what you most need to change in order to lose weight and feel
great. Visit www.patrickholford.com and select the '100% health' tab at the top.

Nutrition clubs
For those of you who would like some moral support and on-the-ground advice
on weight loss on the Holford Low-GL Diet, the Zest4life nutrition clubs are for you.
Zest4life is a health network run by qualifed nutritionists. See www.holforddiet.com
for more information.

Psychocalisthenics
Psychocalisthenics is an excellent exercise system that takes less than 20 minutes
a day, develops strength, suppleness and stamina, and generates vital energy.
The best way to learn it is to do the Psychocalisthenics training courses. See
www.patrickholford.com (Events) for details on these, or call +44 (0)20 8871 2949.
Also available is the book *Master Level Exercise: Psychocalisthenics* and a
Psychocalisthenics CD and DVD. For further information see www.pcals.com.

Food or chemical allergy and intolerance
YorkTest sell a home test kit for food and chemical allergies that requires a
pinprick blood sample. You don't have to go to your doctor. YorkTest laboratories
will test you for sensitivity to all foods including gluten, gliadin, wheat and yeast,

using both IgG ELISA testing and the IgE allergy test. Call YorkTest for a Food Sensitivity Test kit on freephone 0800 074 6185 (UK). Visit www.yorktest.com for more information and prices.

Low-GL food lists

I am constantly assessing the GL content of new foods. Please register with my website www.patrickholford.com or www.holforddiet.com to find up-to-date information about South African, Australian, branded and other foods. You can also refer to my pocket-sized book, *The Holford Diet GL Counter*.

Body-fat percentage scales

These can be purchased from a variety of outlets such as Argos (www.argos.co.uk), Boots (www.boots.com) or websites such as www.scalesexpress.com.

LOW-GL FOODS

Solo Low Sodium Sea Salt

The average person gets far too much sodium because we eat too much salt (sodium chloride) and salted foods, and not enough potassium and magnesium, found in fruits and vegetables. Not all salt, however, is bad for you. Solo Low Sodium Sea Salt contains 60 per cent less sodium and is high in the essential minerals of magnesium and potassium. It is sold in the UK, Ireland, Spain, the Netherlands, Singapore, Hong Kong, Japan, Bahrain, Saudi Arabia, United Arab Emirates, Jordan, the Baltic states and the US. Visit their website www.soloseasalt.com for more information or call +44 (0)845 130 4568.

Xylitol

While it is best to avoid sugar and sugar alternatives as much as possible, there are two natural sugars that have the lowest GL score. These are blue agave syrup, which is used to sweeten healthier drinks, and xylitol. Xylitol is available from Totally Nourish: visit www.totallynourish.com.

Low-GL Get Up & Go

Low-GL Get Up & Go is the perfect Holford Low-GL Diet breakfast – a delicious, creamy superfood smoothie mix, made from powdered wholefoods, which you blend with strawberries and banana. It's available from good health food stores, or from www.totallynourish.com.

INDEX

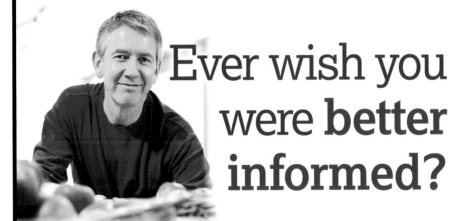

Ever wish you were **better informed?**

Join my 100% Health Club today and you'll receive:

✔ My newsletter, plus Special Reports on vital health topics

✔ Immediate access to hundreds of health articles and special reports.

✔ Have your questions answered in our Members Only blogs.

✔ Save money on supplements, books and other health products.

✔ Save up to £50 on Patrick Holford's **100% Health Workshop**.

✔ Become part of a community of like-minded people and help others.

JOIN TODAY at **www.patrickholford.com**

    Being a member has transformed my life, and that of many of my family and friends. Patrick's information is always spot on and really practical. My member benefits and discounts save me much more than the subscription. Being a member is a must if you want to be and stay healthy.

Joyce Taylor

100%Health®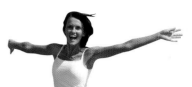

Weekend Intensive

The workshop that works.

Learn how to go from 'average' to superhealthy in a weekend.

Do YOU want to:

✔ Take control of your own health?

✔ Master your weight?

✔ Turn back the clock?

✔ Prevent and reverse disease?

✔ Transform your diet, your health and your life?

Discover the **8 secrets of optimum living** - and put them into action with your own individualised personal health and fitness programme with **Patrick Holford**.

"I thought I was healthy. I feel absolutely fantastic. It's changed my life." Karen S.

"Learnt more in a day than a lifetime. Definitely recommended." *Sarah F.*

"It worked miraculously. I lost 5 stones in 5 months. Life has become very good." *Fiona F.*

"I have so much more energy. I wake up raring to go. It's changed my life." *Matthew F.*

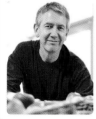

"You can wake up full of energy, with a clear mind and balanced mood, never gain weight and stay disease free. Having worked with over 60,000 people I know what changes are going to most rapidly transform how you feel."
Patrick Holford

"Visionary." *Independent*

"Health guru Patrick Holford addresses the true causes of illness." *Guardian*

"One of the world's leading authorities on new approaches to health" *Daily Mail*

Thousands of people have transformed their health.

Why not become one of them?
Find out more at **www.patrickholford.com**